ONE BRICK

AT A TIME

Breaking Down the Wall of Bitterness
and Learning to Trust God

To Ronald Manton,
Jon Elaine

Elaine Oostra

Copyright 2016 by Elaine Oostra
Published by Field of View Press
Parma, Idaho

Cover designed by Tom Hollis
Edited by Bonnie VanCleave and JoEllen Claypool

I have tried to recreate events, locales and conversations from my memories of them. In order to maintain their anonymity in some instances I have changed the names of individuals and places, along with some identifying characteristics and details such as physical properties, occupations and places of residence.

For more information or additional copies please contact:
Field of View Press
P.O. Box 1087
Parma, Idaho
fieldofviewpress@gmail.com

First printing 2016
ISBN – 978-0-9972316-0-1
Library of Congress Control Number – 2016901941

DEDICATION

I want to dedicate this book to my grandkids and my children and pray for their desire to know God's unconditional love and to know His forgiveness when they cry out and repent. I dedicate this story to those who desire to be overcomers and no longer victims of painful pasts.

"When I kept silent about my sin, my body wasted away through my groaning all day long. For day and night Your hand was heavy upon me; My vitality was drained as with the fever heat of summer. I acknowledged my sin to You, and my iniquity I did not hide; I said, 'I will confess my transgressions to the LORD'; And You forgave the guilt of my sin." (Psalm 32:3-5, New American Standard Bible)

"Let each generation tell its children of your mighty acts; let them proclaim your power." (Psalm 145:4, New Living Translation)

Elaine Oostra

CONTENTS

FOREWORD

Foreword by Barb Ludy

There is nothing that pleases me more than to recommend this book to readers. The author, as a person, is delightful and she writes like she talks. One can almost taste the sadness and delight in each little vignette of life as she poignantly describes it. I've had the wonderful experience of knowing Elaine and watching her passionately invest in lives around her, refusing to take identity in her past. May you be encouraged as you read, because life does have difficulties and overcoming is what is promised to us as we look to the Overcomer. Grab a hot (she loves hot) cup of coffee, your favorite blanky, and curl up on a comfy couch and enjoy!

Foreword by Bonnie VanCleave

I had the privilege of helping Elaine with parts of her book. This paragraph stuck with me: "It was Sunday morning. My dad walked outside and nailed the bedroom window shut. After switching the lock from the inside to the outside of his and Mom's room, he calmly walked over to Mom. Gently picking her up, he carried her, kicking and screaming, into the bedroom. He turned and walked out locking the door behind him. Leaving my brothers at home, Dad and I left for church."

Not your typical Sunday morning. Or was it?

Elaine grew up in a small rural area in northern Washington State, not far from the Canadian border, in the late 1950's. Life was simple in this tiny Dutch community. Dairy farming barely brought in enough money for the family needs, let alone anything extra.

Many struggles plagued Elaine as she grew into womanhood.

Being raised in a loving Christian home did not make it easy, however. Memories of growing up played a unique role in how she viewed God and life. Why did her dad take her and her siblings to neighbors and family members in the middle of the night? Why did her mom suddenly lash out at people? Where did she go? What was this place? Didn't God care? No answers seemed to come.

Eventually, God did answer in a mighty way. But, as in all things, His plan is perfect and is revealed in His time. Elaine has been my close friend for over 10 years. We met at Sterry Memorial Church in Parma, Idaho, both of us finding our way to this small rural community from other areas. Our friendship grew from attending women's retreats, planning church events, and serving on church session together. We have shared a multitude of prayers, laughs, and tears. Most importantly, we share a belief in Jesus Christ our Lord and Savior, who died for our sins.

Elaine Oostra, you are a true sister in Christ. I celebrate your courage for allowing your readers to experience how God grows each of His children in Faith, Hope and Love. "The greatest of these is LOVE." 1 Corinthians 13:13

ACKNOWLEDGMENT

"The living, the living, he thanks You, as I do this day; the father (mother) makes known to the children Your faithfulness." (Isaiah 38:19, English Standard Version)

I want to thank my husband, Ken, who has supported me throughout this process. I appreciate him for allowing me to be transparent even on our personal struggles in our marriage, and what we overcame.

I want to make a tribute to my parents and their marriage and to my dad's faithfulness to my mom. He meant what he said, "In sickness and in health, till death do us part." I saw their love for each other, imperfect as it was and full of many trials and tribulations.

I had amazing and fun women who helped me in editing and encouraged me in this adventure: Barb, Bonnie, and JoEllen.

Thank you to my dear friends, Barb and Bonnie, for writing my foreword.

There were so many times I was doubtful if I should continue writing this book. God has brought confirmation to me in many ways. One example: I needed to find a pair of saddle shoes for my cover picture. I looked in a second-hand store. Nothing. In my car I prayed, "Lord if I am supposed to write and publish this book, could you please confirm to me and help me find saddle shoes, size two. It will be my fleece."

I was about to go home when I passed another second-hand store. I felt a nudge to turn around and go back. I almost talked myself out of it. I headed straight to the shoe racks upon entering the store. Smack dab in in the middle of all these dark shoes I see white and black saddle shoes! I do a lot of second-hand store shopping and have never seen these there. I raced over to them, afraid someone else might want the treasure I spotted. I picked them up. Yes, they were a size two! Wow, God, You did it! Thank you Jesus, my Savior!

Elaine Oostra

INTRODUCTION

My husband Ken has encouraged me many times that I have a story to tell. This is my story.

I believed the lie for years that I was the only one who felt or did certain things that I write about. I know now there are more people like me. We, as humans, are not that unique. *"There is nothing new under the sun."* **(Ecclesiastes 1:9b.)**

I have learned, in talking with other women, that we have a common thread. We hide things that we think others will not accept about us. Rejection is a big fear. Until we are secure in our relationship with Christ, we struggle with the fear of acceptance. The enemy loves to keep us silent and alone.

God will continue to shelter you and me, if we humble ourselves before Him and seek righteousness according to Zephaniah 2:3. It's His promise. I am amazed at how God is faithful and has heard the cry of my heart and what God has healed in me. I see God's hand everywhere, in all areas of my life!

Each of my siblings could write their own story according to their own unique point of view. In birth order I was number two, the first girl by God's design. Mental illness was very much a part of our lives growing up. Each member of my family handled it differently. Learning to respect this in each other has come with its own challenges.

I want to help people understand the depression/ schizophrenia that plagued my mother and my eldest brother without going into much detail of what they did personally in their behaviors. Learning about this illness has also been healing to me. It helps me to feel, well, maybe normal because many times you don't when things seem out of control. I am no expert of this illness. I can only share what I do know and what I've experienced.

1
SCARED LITTLE GIRL

"Can you take the kids again? I need to take my wife to the hospital," my dad asked with a baby in his arms and three frightened little ones hanging on his pant legs. He stood on the porch steps of the adjacent neighboring farmhouse, tears in his eyes, and at a loss as to what to do.

I lay alone in bed in the upstairs room of the neighbor's house, sobbing hard with my face buried in the pillow so no one would hear me, "I want my daddy, and I want to go home!" Lifting my head from the pillow, wet with tears, I heard the two teenage boys that shared a room down the hall talking. I didn't want them to know I was crying. Wiping my face off with the sheet, struggling to stop crying, I sat on the edge of the bed and planned my escape. At the end of the hall was a window above the front porch roof. My five-year-old brain thought I could open the window, crawl onto the roof, slide down the poles, and run home, but I was too scared. I was very homesick, even though I was only a field length away from home.

Sometimes, I shared the bed with the eldest daughter of the home. I would wake up, barely hanging on to the edge of the bed. She was not used to sharing. I liked it when she was home from college; I didn't feel so lonely. She was kind to me and made me feel happy when I was so sad.

I am thankful for our neighbors who took us in. They were older than my parents, very strict and went to the same church that we did. I did like the father of the home, a friend of my dad's. He had a kindness that drew me to him. He would sit in the covered porch area before or after milking cows. There were homemade, small, bean-filled bags, toy wagons and tractors that I would play with while he smiled down at me and talked with me sometimes. His wife was always busy in the kitchen. After dinner, he would read the Bible. I would watch the white and black cat clock ticking loudly above the table with its big eyes and tail swaying opposite of each other, back and forth. As predictable as that cat clock, so was the father of the home just as predictable at falling asleep in the middle of reading the Bible or praying. I would silently giggle as his wife would call out his name and nudge him awake.

About a mile down the road was another sweet, elderly, couple that would take us for short stays until we went to other homes. The wife was always smiling and happy. She had a Dutch accent, was short, a little stocky and big breasted (*when I was little, they were my pillows that I would rest my head upon*) like my grandmother. I felt loved there. To make us feel better, they gave us pink and white peppermints.

It's funny to me the little things I remembered as I started my healing journey.

2
THE OLD FARMHOUSE

The two-story farmhouse my grandfather built is where I recall some of my earliest memories of my mother's illness. I was starting to see something was not right.

The incident is still vivid in my mind. Our family hosted a young man who was part of an out-of-state choir that our church sponsored. The young man was sitting in the big, green, arm chair blowing up balloons in the front room. He rubbed them on his head, making his hair stand on end, all the while entertaining us kids in the room. I was jumping up and down, giggling with delight watching his hair fly and the balloons stick to the mirror on the wall behind the chair.

Suddenly, the mood changed. My mother angrily entered the room and grabbed the balloons. "Stop that!" she yelled. I stood there frozen, my eyes wide and full of fear. I was so ashamed of my mom and embarrassed for this young man who was not sure what to do. We all were sent to our rooms because mom wanted to sleep, something she did a lot. I didn't understand why she acted this way.

There was the manic side of mental illness and on the flip side was the depression. The depression would make my mom want to sleep a lot or hide away.

In this old house, there was a back porch with no lock on the back door. In order to lock it, my mom would take a butter knife and lodge it in between the door jam and the door. This way she could lock me and my siblings outside so she could sleep. I did not even think this was unusual until I had my own kids. I could not lock my kids out of the house and sleep peacefully like my mother would. However, as a child, to me this was normal.

It became a game to shake the door knob until the knife fell out. When my mom would hear the knife fall, she would yell at us then put the knife back in. We would do it again, more quietly, and sneak into the freezer on the back porch, steal frozen applesauce and spoons, then escape to the fort my big brother had built in the huge apple tree out back. Up in the fort, sin was delicious! Scraping the frozen crystals of applesauce from the plastic containers, we giggled at conquering the "knife in the door".

3
FIRE!

One Sunday morning, while our family was sitting in church, the town's fire alarm blew loudly, interrupting the pastor's sermon. A man ran frantically into the church to our pew row and whispered to my dad. My dad had a very serious look on his face. He left hurriedly with the man and said nothing to my mom or us kids. It did not occur to my 8-year-old mind that the fire siren was for our home. As a young child, you don't think about things like that. It was always other people's homes.

That was the day our old farmhouse burned beyond repair. My older brother had wanted to stay home from church that day, but my dad insisted that he was to go. God knew he was not to be there that day.

After church, I saw my mom talking with other women, a worried look on her face. Through her tears, she was asking about the piano. It hit me then that it was our home. My mom treasured that piano. She had picked raspberries to buy it. It cost $100. That was a lot of money and many hours in the raspberry patch. My mom worked very hard. Every day for three weeks, we went with Mom to the raspberry patch to help. That piano cost my mom over 1200 flats of raspberries! The thought of it being burned up was devastating. We found out later that the soundboard cracked from the heat of the fire. We still were able to use it for piano lessons, even though it was always out of tune.

As my siblings and I were sent to the homes of friends, someone took my mom to see the damage. The people I stayed with drove me by the house. It was unbelievable. Our home was gone. We could no longer live there.

The owner of the raspberry patch had a house by the river. We called it the workers' house. People would stay there for the summer to work in the raspberries. Berry season was over and the house was vacant; we moved in. I hated it. It was so ugly and void of everything I was familiar with. I was embarrassed that we had to live there. All of us kids slept in the same bedroom downstairs. We didn't go upstairs often because of the pornographic posters taped on the wall by the people who lived there during the summer.

Shortly after we moved into the workers' house, my dad started building our new home with the help of our neighbors, church friends, and family. It was a very basic, ranch-style home with plywood floors minus a completed bathroom and all of the inside doors. The funds were not there to finish the house. There was a small bathroom in the garage where my dad cleaned up after working in the barn. He built and plumbed a cement shower. There was also a sink and a toilet. We used this bathroom for many years. The extended family did gather money together so there would be linoleum on the kitchen floor.

Living in a stressful situation can change the dynamics in a family. While living in the workers' house, we all got the measles at the same time. As the holidays approached, all of the responsibilities and the expectations placed upon my mom may have been too much. Once again, Dad had to take Mom to the mental hospital. It was a hard time. I didn't have to stay with the neighbors this time. At nine years old, I was left in charge.

Meals were provided by the church women. One meal brought to us was a potato casserole with hot dogs in it. It was my responsibility to make sure everybody ate because my dad had to go milk cows at our dairy and it would be late before he got home. While washing the dishes, I barfed up the hot dogs and potatoes. Thinking I was dying I called my dad at the dairy barn and told him I got sick. Stopping the milking process and rushing the mile home, my dad arrived and determined I had eaten too fast. Maybe I did, I don't know. I just remember feeling so bad that my dad had to leave the cows to clean up my mess. He was not happy with me.

We had a family dog we loved very much. One day we found it dead on the road. We cried and cried. This was just another tragedy to add to the stresses our family was dealing with. Our aunt and uncle brought us a new puppy. I think they did this to cheer us up while we lived in this house that was not our true home and our mom was in the hospital. It diverted our attention off the circumstances around us. The puppy cried so much the first few nights that my dad placed it in a box and put him in the back seat of our tan Oldsmobile so my dad couldn't hear him. That way he didn't get cold. We named the black puppy Blacky. We had him for many years. I remember dressing Blacky in clothes as well as our kitties.

We finally got to move into our new home that spring. The room that was to be a bathroom became our play room. We would play school. When I was in the seventh grade, I did my science fair project in there. I had seeds growing in a cardboard box. My project showed the need for good soil and watering. I won second place in the science fair! I couldn't believe it when the science teacher told me. I was told the judges wanted to give me first place, but my project would not last until the next competition. I didn't care. I had won! I never won a prize in school.

I think my dad finally finished the bathroom in the house when I was in the eighth grade. If someone were to remodel that bathroom, they would see our years of drawing and writing behind the walls. My room never did get closet doors; only one bedroom got them. We did get doors to the bedrooms and red carpet for the front room a few years after moving in. I don't remember when we got carpet in the bedrooms. It never bothered me that it took so long to finish the home. We never had a lot. My dad always knew to the penny how much money he had in his wallet. I found this out the hard way.

We lived less than a mile from the town store and the town park. I loved black licorice and wanted some badly. I went into my parents' bedroom and saw my dad's wallet on the dresser. I knew it was wrong, but I opened it anyway and saw a few coins. I thought I would just take a quarter since there were two; my dad might not notice one was missing. I talked my brother into walking to town with me to go and play at the park. Mom was going to pick us up later. I told him to play while I went to the store a block away.

Licorice was one cent a piece which meant I was able to buy twenty five pieces. I had never had so much licorice! I was happy as I walked back to the park with my bag full, until I saw our car driving up to the park, *Oh no, what am I going to do with all this licorice!* I thought. I finally realized what I had done. I panicked as I looked around, wondering where I could hide it. I had to get rid of it fast. My mom was telling us to get in the car.

There were kids on the merry-go-round. "Here, you guys, want some candy?" I asked them all and handed it out as fast as I could. I didn't even get one piece. That night at the dinner table, Dad asked us kids if any of us had taken a quarter out of his wallet. I am sure guilt was all over my face, but I never did tell my dad that I took it; I felt guilty. My dad worked so hard. He didn't even have enough money to do the finishing touches on our new home and replace items lost in the fire. Times were hard then; every coin mattered. I never stole from my dad's wallet again.

4

PAIN

My body broke into convulsive crying. I could no longer hold in all the painful emotions and anxiety I had. It was too much for me to bear. I was sitting in church next to my dad, recalling the morning's events. The lady behind me touched my back. My dad handed me his hankie and asked me if I wanted to go home. "No, Daddy!" I said, still crying. I really didn't want to go home, so I made myself stop.

That morning before church, my dad got some nails and a hammer. I watched anxiously as he nailed the bedroom window shut. He then took off the bedroom door knob and put the lock on so that it faced the outside. Mom was not taking her medication and was too unpredictable and manic.

The state's mandates would not allow my dad to commit her to the mental hospital she normally went to when she was sick. She had not hurt us or herself yet. There were times we couldn't find her and the police had to search for her. We were always afraid of what the voices in Mom's head would tell her to do.

My dad calmly picked up my mom, who was kicking and screaming, and carried her into the bedroom. It was not a pleasant scene. I even asked my dad if he really had to do that. As he looked at me, I already knew the answer. We left with the sound of my mom banging on the bedroom door. My other siblings stayed home at Dad's request to watch over Mom, with my older brother in charge.

When Dad and I arrived home from church, I could no longer hear the banging and screaming that invaded my ears when we had left. As I walked into the house, my sister and brothers were in their rooms. It was as if nothing out of the ordinary had happened that morning. Dad quietly unlocked the bedroom door and opened it.

There, lying peacefully on the bed, my mother slept, exhausted from the fear-filled screams. Leaving the door ajar, he put on a big can of soup for us. After heating it up, my dad prayed as he always did before each meal. We sat in silence around the kitchen table and reflected on our own thoughts of the events of the morning. One question lingered in my mind: what will Mom do when she wakes up?

I didn't blame him for how he handled this, or wonder why we didn't stay home. It was Sunday; my dad always went to church.

My dad was a farmer and he did not have the skills or education to deal with a mentally ill wife, yet he was expected to. It was exasperating at times. It was difficult for my dad to commit Mom to the mental hospital or to even get her help. It was help that she didn't think she needed when ill. The legislative intent of the 1967 Lanterman-Petris-Short Act was to end the inappropriate, indefinite, and involuntary commitment of a mentally disorderly person. To put it simply, it was thought to be inhuman to lock up mentally ill people and violate their rights. In 1969-70, deinstitutionalization was based on the principle that severe mental illness should be treated in the least restrictive setting.

This all came about because there was abuse in some mental hospitals and people were committed who never should have been committed. However, today the pendulum has swung way too far in the opposite direction. Our laws are now designed to protect individuals from being held against their will, if they suffer from mental illness. This is so they can have a degree of freedom, dignity, and integrity of the body, mind, and spirit. As a result, however, many of them live on the streets or are put in jail. Family members struggle to learn how to live with them. If the mentally ill are on medication and it has taken effect, this would be great but meanwhile, they live in a world of their own where their minds are not well.

It's funny, but not really; we don't ask people with cancer to wait until they are almost dead before they seek treatment. A mentally ill person has to hurt someone or themselves before the law will step in to help. We were told this over and over again. I still feel the anxiety in my heart as I write this regarding what we faced day after day when Mom was ill. It was such a helpless feeling.

This is another Sunday memory. After church my dad would pick us kids up from the different homes in which we were staying. He would take us to see our mom at the hospital. I wanted to see my dad and my mom; I just didn't like going there.

The drive was about 30 miles but felt like it took forever. I was glad to see my siblings. I missed them a lot! When Dad pulled up to the hospital, I wondered what Mom was going to be like. *I don't like this place*, I thought. We walked through the hallway to our mom's room, staring at the patients along the way. I stuck very close to my dad. Mom's thin body was slumped on the edge of her hospital bed, staring at the floor. She did not look up most times that we came.

"Hi Mom." There was no reply back. I said it again. Nothing. She just rocked back and forth. Her hair, normally curled, was flat to her head. *Why won't she talk to me?* I didn't like Mom this way. I wanted to escape.

We left Dad to visit with Mom and went to a familiar spot. In the center of the hospital, near the gift shop, was a banana tree surrounded by a two-foot, circular, brick wall. It's not really normal to have a banana tree in Washington State and yet it was the one place in the mental hospital that felt sane. The people in and around the gift shop weren't as scary as the residents who roamed the hallway.

The banana tree reached toward the sunlight radiating through the glass dome above. Planted around the tree were orchids, azaleas and other colorful flowers. It felt safe for me there, in this place of craziness. The banana tree didn't belong there, any more than I felt I did. We would sit on the short brick wall that surrounded the tree and look up at the glass ceiling in awe. As the brick wall protected the banana tree, I was building a wall of protection without being aware.

I don't remember a lot of the emotions I felt as a little girl around my mom. All I do remember is saying hi and not wanting to be with my mom. She was a stranger who stared into nothingness. Sometimes she would look up and just stare. I wanted her to acknowledge me, maybe tell me she missed me. I missed her! But I got nothing.

After the federal government closed the hospital in the 70's, the greenhouse moved to the state capital gardens in Olympia, Washington along with the banana tree. For some silly reason, I was glad the banana tree had a home.

The drive back home was always hard. We really wouldn't be going back home, but to our "temporary homes." By the time I was in fourth grade, we no longer had to stay with the neighbors when Mom was hospitalized. We were able to be home with Dad.

I found letters in a box full of my mom's saved memories. I remember writing this letter sitting at the kitchen table before my dad left to visit my mom.

It's so hard for me to remember missing her, but I know I did. I wrote it to her. I know something in me shut down at some point in my life to be able to handle her being gone. It felt like forever when I was little and our home was void of Mom.

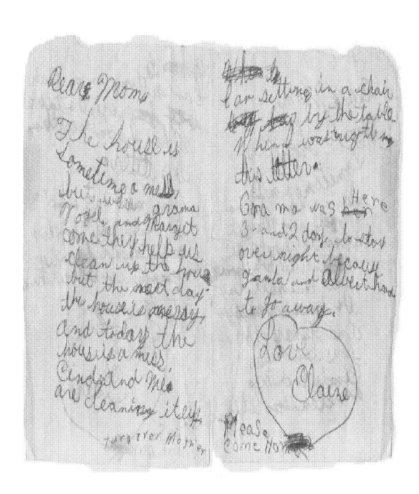

Dear Mom,

    The house is sometimes a mess, but grama Vogel and Margret come they help us clean up the house but the next day the house is messy and today the house is a mess. Cindy and me are cleaning it up. (Turn over Mother) I am sitting in a chair by the table when I was writing this letter. Grama was here 3 and 2 day to stay over night because grandpa and Albert have to go away. Love Elaine Please come home.

Elaine Oostra

5
WALL OF PROTECTION GROWING

I don't care anymore, I give up. I am a failure, I thought to myself sitting on the school bus. I stared out the window, mesmerized at the green farm fields as they fluttered by. It looked like an old movie screen with the telephone poles along the road seemingly marking each film clip. It helped me forget the humiliation I knew that I was about to face.

My dad had called me into the kitchen earlier that summer and told me the worst news a fourth grader could receive. "Elaine, you are failing fourth grade and the teacher wants you to do it over." I stood there in disbelief.

"No, they can't do that; I won't go back to school!" I cried out. My world instantly crumbled before me. I thought my life was over, my summer was ruined! Everyone would know. They would laugh at me when I went back.

The summer ended. My dreaded day came. The bus pulled up to the elementary school. My heart pounded in my chest. Fear engulfed me. I got off the bus, waiting for the kids to notice, wishing I could be invisible. Walking toward the school I heard my classmates yell out the school bus windows, "Elaine, you are not supposed to get off here. We are going to the middle school now!"

What I dreaded all summer came true. One kid had figured it out. "She failed. That's why she got off the bus," he yelled out as others joined him, "She failed!"

Humiliation and tears came. Their words confirmed to me what I already felt about myself.

I walked into the familiar hallway. I turned and watched the bus pull away with my best friends on their way to the middle school. I hung up my school bag, out of habit, on last year's hook. A fourth grade girl came up to me, "Didn't you do fourth grade last year?" she asked. I just wanted to die. I felt like God didn't care about me. He cared about others more.

At recess time, I sat pressed up against the corner wall outside the fourth grade classroom with my knees pulled up to my chest. I pulled my gray skirt over my knees covering my gray cable knit tights that matched my gray sweater. I wrapped my arms around my legs and stared down at my black and white saddle shoes. I wanted to hide. The color of my outfit matched my dismal mood. My blond, shoulder-length hair fell forward to cover my face. I peeked up and looked through the strands of hair and saw my classmates playing on the playground. I was filled with fear and shame, yet a part of me wanted to join them.

I wish I could say things changed the next year. I remember myself standing up against the big green school doors, hidden under the archway. That day I just wanted to be left alone. My arms were protectively wrapped tightly around my chest, watching the kids play, hoping that no one would see me. *I wish I was invisible. I hate fifth grade. I hate school!* Since I had to do fourth grade twice, my best friends were in sixth grade and had different recess time. I had no friends. I tried to make new ones, only to be rejected.

A classmate ran up to me and asked what was wrong. "My mom is in the hospital," I said.

"Why?" she asked.

"Um, um, she is sick," I replied back quickly with fear. *Why did I say that?* I thought to myself. My heart started racing as I stood looking like a cat that just got dunked in a tub of water. I was angry at myself. Thoughts flashed through my mind. *What if she would ask more questions? What would I say? I couldn't tell her my mom was in a mental hospital. I couldn't! How would I explain that? What would that say about me? Oh please, leave me alone!* Thankfully, she walked away. Deep inside, I wanted to tell someone, but who could I tell?

A thought came to me. Since she talked to me, just maybe she would be my friend. I saw she was with another girl and I followed them out to the ball field. The other girl turned around and said sarcastically, "Stop following us. You are not our friend."

I froze in my tracks, rejected and speechless. I turned around with my head down and headed back to the big green doors with shame and humiliation once again.

It's funny the memories that stay with us from childhood, yet others are so long forgotten. I can still see in my mind the young, scared girl. I want to run to this little girl in my memories. I know all the trials and tribulations she will be going through. I want to hold her like I do my grandbabies and reassure her that God has His hand on her life.

I had a hard time concentrating in school. Sometimes when the teacher was talking, I couldn't hear or understand what she said. My mind may have still been on whatever happened the night before, or that very morning, or what would await me when I got home after school with my mom's unpredictable behavior. I fell more and more behind in learning. Somehow, in my immature, young mind, I felt responsible for taking care of the home. My dad, in later years, told me he felt I had had too much responsibility handed to me being the oldest girl. What happens in a home very much affects a child's ability to learn, each child handling things differently according to their personality and each being impacted in a different way.

Elaine Oostra

6
GLIMPSES OF GOD'S LOVE

Every Memorial Day, our family, including cousins, aunts, and uncles, would go to Canada and have a picnic in a park near Harrison Hot Springs. Before we went to the indoor pool, everyone would hike up to the source of the natural hot springs and watch the steaming hot water bubble out of the ground. When the food would settle, we would all head over to the hot springs pool. This was one of the highlights of my growing up years that I looked forward to with great anticipation.

I desperately needed a new bathing suit. My mom ordered my very first two-piece piece bathing suit from the Sears Catalog. It was yellow with little white flowers. The top part had an apron that was detachable and covered my stomach.

Memorial Day was fast approaching and my suit had not yet come in the mail. I had nothing to wear if that swimsuit didn't come. I wouldn't be able to swim with my cousins. It was Saturday, my last chance. There was no mail on Sunday and the coming Monday was Memorial Day. No mail! *God please let my swimsuit be in the mail. Show me You love me! Please let it be in there!* I prayed as I walked across the country road to our metal mailbox. It sat on a wooden post at the edge of the small ditch which was filled with tall blades of sharp green grass. A yellow finch was sitting nearby singing. I stood in front of the mailbox saying out loud, "Show me, God, that You are real and care."

I opened the mailbox. I couldn't believe it! There it was, a brown paper package with Sears writing on it! I ripped the package open and pulled out my yellow bathing suit. With tears of happiness, I felt God's love for me. He really cared about me, even in the midst of unpredictable chaos in my young life.

Why didn't moments and memories like this assure me forever of God's love? Maybe you, like me, forget so fast when God reassures us of His love.

7
MIXTURE OF FOND CHILDHOOD MEMORIES

Pleasant memories can get pushed into the background of our minds when we only focus on the harshness of life. When I really learned to trust God, these pleasant memories were unleashed and they overpowered the unpleasant ones. I would like to share some of the fond recollections I have that spanned across the years of my childhood.

THE RIVER

I grew up in a small rural area on a dairy farm that my father had purchased from his father. It was nestled up against the backdrop of the Nooksack Mountains in Northwest Washington.

My dad loved to hike in the mountains and hills a couple of miles behind our home. It was like entering another world, a peaceful world. Sometimes, I would go with my friends and my dad. I loved having this time with him. It made me feel as if we had a 'normal' family.

One particularly hot summer day, Dad took my friend and me up the mountain. He was way ahead of us. "I am so hot." I said to my friend. "Let's take our shirts off. No one is up here."

We giggled and dared each other. We were thirteen and still very self-conscious of our bodies. We didn't get far down the path, shirtless, when we looked up and saw a man hiking toward us on our trail. We took the shirts, which were tied around our waists, and put them on as quickly as we could, giggling the whole time.

Years later, my dad shared this passion of hiking with my oldest daughter. I believe this helped him to cope with the craziness.

"I lift my eyes up to the hills. From where does my help come? My help comes from the LORD who made heaven and earth." (Psalm 121:1-2, ESV)

Springtime would often bring the melting snows gushing down the mountains into the river that shared its name. This river bordered my dad's farmland and would flood the lower and upper fields in front of our house. The brown river water would inch its way across the road daring you to stop it. Soon the farm would be surrounded by flowing water within a matter of a few hours or less. In the old farmhouse, it would come onto the porch but never into the house.

I remember in the new farmhouse, the river would threaten to come in the front door but never did. Because the garage was lower than the house, my dad would open the garage doors and the back door to the garage and let the river flow through. My dad kind of liked this because the river would clean out the barn and barnyard. My dad always saw positive in every situation.

SILAGE TRUCK

My dad would take us kids on simple day trips just to get us out of the house when my mom wasn't doing well. Those day trips were fond memories. I remember the trips to pick up pea silage. We would all sit next to Dad on the bench seat of the old, stick-shift farm truck and watch the road go by through a hole in the floor boards. When the truck was being loaded up with silage, I would sit on the top of the truck with one of my brothers and suck on the pea pods. They were full of flavor. The fermentation made them taste sour, but they were "yummy" to us. On the way home we would stop at a honey stand and buy fresh honey. That honey stand is still there today. We looked forward to those times with our dad.

HIKING

My dad enjoyed sharing his love for hiking with us. He would take us on many adventures I thought unknown to man. Nothing could get in my dad's way. Not even roaring waters gushing down the mountain would keep us from crossing. We walked until dad would spot a fallen tree over the wild creek. Fear never seemed to enter my dad's mind. It did mine!

When I saw an obstacle in front of me, my dad seemed to see a challenge in front of him. I would watch my dad. I could see his mind turning as he talked to himself. I knew he was going to make us go over those logs to get to the other side. I was terrified. *I am going to do this afraid or not*, I thought to myself. I didn't want to disappoint my dad. I also trusted him. If he felt we could do this, then we could, and we did!

Today I have this same mindset I learned from my dad when things look impossible. If there is a will, then there is a way. I do see difficulties as a challenge to overcome; in my childhood, I saw them as obstacles to stop me.

"¹⁰ **but when the perfect comes, the partial will pass away. ¹¹ When I was a child, I spoke like a child, I thought like a child, I reasoned like a child. When I became a man, I gave up childish ways. ¹² For now we see in a mirror dimly, but then face to face. Now I know in part; then I shall know fully, even as I have been fully known." (I Corinthians 13:10-12, ESV)**

My dad was not a man of words or physical affection. I don't remember him saying, "I love you," but I always knew he did. It was in his actions. He worked hard and didn't spend money frivolously, except for our private education and Mom's medical bills. He read the Bible and prayed at each meal. Church attendance was important to him. I could see he had a relationship with Jesus. He modeled to me what it meant to have freedom in Christ. My mom was raised in a strict Christian home. She thought we shouldn't ride our bikes on Sunday, but Dad would let us.

BLACK AND WHITE TV

"Good morning, boys and girls," the children's TV character said, "I see you sitting in front of the TV in your pajamas."

As a young girl, I thought he could really see me. This is the one entertainment we had. Like most people in that era, it was a big-boxed, black and white TV with only one or two channels.

When I got a little older, I moved on from kids' shows to the Sunday night TV movies. The problem was, we didn't get that channel so we would go to the neighbor's and watch the movie through their front window. Sometimes we were invited in and would lay on the floor in front of their color TV. It was the highlight of my week.

BACKYARD APPLE TREE

My brothers and I made tents under the apple tree with stinky, black plastic that my dad used to cover the grass silage. We would put old wood furniture in it and pretend it was our house. We discovered the pincher bugs would invade the tent during the night. It creeps me out to think we could have spent the night with earwigs crawling all over us. Sometimes we would use my grandpa's old paint tarps and drape them over the clothesline.

My oldest brother and I brought empty milk cartons home from school and would take them up to our fort in the apple tree. We created little houses from the cartons, attempting to glue them together with a mixture of flour and water. I think we had more glue mix on ourselves than on the makeshift houses we tried to create.

"I will always protect you from any bullies at school," my brother said to me up in the tree.

I remember it made me feel good to know that. I believed him. He was my protector. I miss who he was then. As he grew older, the mental illness he had changed him. It invaded his mind when he was a teenager.

BARN

Because we didn't have a lot of toys, we spent our summers playing outside. I don't remember being in the house much. My siblings and the neighbor kids would build forts in the haymow, even when we were told not to. We would make tunnels with the hay bales that led to a bigger room. I think these would cave in when my dad had to feed the cows. Maybe he fell through our makeshift roofs.

Our grandfather had a barn also where we would play with our cousins. At one end of this old barn, where the hay was stored, was a loft. From a big log beam high in the arch of the ceiling hung a thick rope. Whenever we went to our grandparents' house, we would race out to the barn to go and swing. One of us would stay down below the loft and swing the rope up to the rest of us to catch it. The big knot on the end of the rope was the seat. We would fight to see who would get to go first.

I have wonderful memories of sitting on that big knot with my heart pounding in my chest. Lifting my feet up from the loft floor, I went flying across the length of the barn. The goal was to swing back to the loft by using my feet to push off from the opposite barn wall. These old barns are a rarity today. Some that are still around are being restored as landmarks. I wonder how many kids today play in barns as we used to do. Barn swings are probably illegal to even have like we had. This kind of makes me sad.

WOODS AND NEIGHBORS

The wooded area that lined the river was only a field away from our house and extended our playground. It was the perfect place to make huts with tree limbs that had broken off in the windstorms. The neighbors would go with us to build huts with the limbs. Someone came up with the great idea of making a campfire. The neighbor boy happened to have matches in his pocket. We got a good roaring fire going and were so proud of ourselves.

"Shhh, I hear yelling," I said.

"Oh no, it's my dad!" shouted the neighbor boy. His dad came running through the field toward us. He was yelling with his arms flailing over his head. Was he ever mad. Furious would be a better word.

"You g-- damn kids! What do you think you are doing? Are you trying to burn down the whole g--damn woods!" he yelled at us. "I am going to wring your necks," was his favorite thing to say. I had never heard my dad swear, so I wondered if God would strike my neighbor's dad dead with lightning.

I always would think and wonder how he would put a ring around our necks. He stomped on our fire that we had worked on so hard. "You kids get home right now and don't you come down here again!" But we did, when he was at work. Back then we were naughty, but we had no fear of him.

He was a painter and kept all his supplies in his garage. Even though he locked it, we would get in many times. There were boxes of sparkles that drew us in. The neighbor boy's dad used them to spray on house ceilings but we had other ideas. We would go in there and throw the sparkles around; it was so pretty watching the sparkly things float down. We would dance around and let the sparkles fall on us. Consequently, we were threatened again to get our necks wrung.

NEIGHBOR'S TREE FORT

Most of my childhood was spent playing with the neighbor kids. They were third or fourth cousins. We could easily walk to their house less than a fourth of a mile away. They had a tree fort too in which we played. On one occasion, the tree fort was getting crowded with all of the kids piled into it. I thought I would go out on a branch and see how far I could go. The ground was maybe 10 feet or more from where I was.

"Elaine, don't go out that far!" the kids yelled at me.

"I am OK," I said back.

Crack! I heard it with no time to react. When I came to, all I could do was moan. The pain hit me hard. The kids were circled around me just laughing. I guess I was making funny faces in my pain.

My brother ran home to get Mom instead of going to the neighbor's house in whose yard I had landed. Mom drove up at the same time the neighbor lady came out yelling, "Why didn't you kids get me?"

My mom tried to pick me up and make me walk while she held onto me. I cried out in pain as she lay me in the back seat of the car and took me to the doctor's office in town. They put me on a stretcher so I didn't have to walk. The X-ray showed I had a cracked hip bone. I had to lie in bed, flat on my back, for a full week. You can't cast a hip. For an eleven year old who is used to being outside, this was like a jail sentence. The worst part was I had to use a bedpan! When the week was over, I used crutches for another week.

GOOD CHRISTMAS MEMORIES

There were happy times when we went to my grandparents' house for Christmas. Sometimes the snow drifts were six feet or higher along the sides of the road from the northeastern winter winds. My dad would wrap blankets around us to keep us warm in the back of the canopy-covered pickup. As a kid, this was an adventure to me. We would giggle at the puffs of air, watching them turn into white mists of crystals. Peering through the canopy window, the walls of snow made it seem as if we were going through a tunnel.

The excitement of being with my cousins, aunts, and uncles

still fills my mind with wonderful memories. I can still see my aunt playing the old pump organ that came on the boat when my mom and her family emigrated from Holland in 1949. We would all gather around the organ and sing hymns and Christmas carols.

My grandparents had a live Christmas tree. Mom didn't believe in Christmas trees. We never had one growing up. As kids, we wanted a tree so badly. We would make our own out of cardboard and color it with decorations, prop it up in the corner and put our one present a piece under it. After we all left the nest, Mom changed her mind and got an artificial tree.

When mom was well, life was pretty much normal for us. My mom had a quiet personality and didn't interact with us a lot. She did take care of our basic needs. When Dad wasn't around, we could always talk Mom into letting us do whatever Dad wouldn't let us do.

One fond memory I have is sitting by Mom with my siblings as she would read us a Bible story before we went to bed. She also taught me to bake, cook, can food, and clean. Baking pies, bars, breads, and cookies was something Mom was very good at. She made the most perfect pie crust, something I never achieved, even though I had her teach me how. I just didn't have the baking touch like she did. My mom's lemon pies have been the family's favorite and always the request for any get together through all the years and times my mom was able to bake.

I do recall times when Mom was happy. She would dance! The record player filled the front room with lively gospel songs as Mom would twirl around and giggle. It would embarrass me. I was not used to seeing my mom happy like this. I would tell her to stop. I didn't know if she was acting normal or not. I didn't know mothers danced like that. I wish now I would have danced with her.

8
MEMORIES NOT AS PLEASANT

As I look back on my childhood, I have wonderful memories mixed with very difficult ones.

Because we attended church, we had different pastors come over and try to talk my mom out of her illness. They would sit on the couch with her and Dad. I would hear them pray for her and read the Bible to her. As kids, we were used to them coming. It was so silly to me what they were trying to do. I remember hiding behind the kitchen wall and peeking around the corner thinking I was sneaky. I would watch and listen to them try and fix her. She never would respond to anything they had to say. Sometimes she would say, "You think I am crazy, don't you?" I would giggle, giving away my hiding spot and be told by my dad to get back into bed.

Some would say my mom had demons and they would try and get the demons out by praying over her. Even as an adult now, I have been told it could have been demon possession. I tell them, "I didn't know you could get a prescription to cure demon possession at the drug store, prescribed by a doctor." When my mom is on her medication regularly, she does not act the same as when she is off it. If it was demon possession, I highly doubt the pills would work. Do I believe there are people out there that may have the same actions as my mom and be possessed? Yes, I do. There is a stigma attached to mental illness. Other illnesses, such as cancer or diabetes, don't carry the same stigma. This is why I didn't talk to anyone and kept it hidden as much as I could.

My mother's mental illness was as predictable as the changing of the seasons each year. Many Thanksgivings and Christmases, Mom would be ill or in the hospital, making holidays difficult.

If Mom was in the hospital, we would not be together as a family. When we were younger, Christmas would be spent with the families with whom we were staying. My younger siblings got to stay with our grandparents. Maybe because I was one the oldest, I was sent to the neighbors.

When I was seven and staying again with neighbors, they gave me a doll. I was so sad that I couldn't even enjoy it. I had tried to talk my little sister into coming and spending Christmas with me, but she wanted to stay at Grandma's. I wanted to go to Grandma's too. Grandma's house was full of love, warmth and family. I sat facing the tree with my new doll. I didn't want to turn around for fear they would see my tears. I didn't want to appear ungrateful for my gift. I thought it was so unfair that the doll for my sister sat under the tree, untouched, but she did not want to come.

One Christmas when Mom was sick, Dad had bought four little boxes of connecting blocks in the gift shop at the mental hospital. I had seen them there while he was visiting Mom. "This is all we get, Dad?" I remember saying. Sometimes there wasn't any money for presents or Dad really didn't have the time to buy gifts. My dad had even taken the time to wrap them. When we opened them, we knew where they came from. Disappointment filled our faces. My poor dad. I didn't even appreciate that he had gotten me a gift.

At the age of 13, I wanted to go shopping. I called my aunt and asked her if she would take my mom, my sister, and me. I loved being with my cousins. She asked me how Mom was doing. To convince my aunt, I lied and told her Mom was doing really well. I justified in my head that everything would be fine. My aunt was unconvinced so I pleaded with her more. I probably threatened my mom to behave herself. I did not want her to ruin our outing.

It was a disaster of an evening! I don't remember any details; they are blocked from my conscience. I just know it did not go well. I was so mad at my mom for ruining the evening. The car ride home from shopping that night was miserable. I was sitting in the back seat of my aunt's car. She turned around, "You said your Mom was fine and she is not." I felt horrible.

My mom's behavior confused me. I had allowed this along with other difficult circumstances to discolor my life. I became bitter.

Elaine Oostra

9
TEENAGER

As my teenage years came upon me, I became angrier at God. Rebellion set in. Teenagers are normally ashamed of their parents to some point. I was extremely embarrassed by my mom when she was ill. Her behavior was unpredictable. You never knew what she would say. She might have felt the need to tell someone off. This is one of the many stages of this particular mental illness.

One day when I was riding home on the school bus, there was my mom walking down the road. She was in her bathrobe with uncombed hair. All the kids could see her from the bus windows. "Who is that?" I heard them say. I thought, *My secret is out.* This was the last thing I wanted.

I was fully aware at this point in my life that our family was not like other families. I resented her and wondered why she just didn't stop doing and saying the things she did when she was ill. It angered and frustrated me. I felt like I hated her.

As a family, we never really talked about how this was affecting each of us. We just lived with it and dealt with it on our own, many times in unhealthy ways. I had no tools to handle it any differently. I was at a loss as to what was happening to my mom. It was just "mental illness" with no real knowledge of the why, just the stigma of "being crazy." I really believed, as a teen, we were the only family in our community that had to deal with this. This brought great shame in my life. I learned in later years about two other families in our church that had fathers with mental illness. Perhaps if I had known of this then, the stigma I had lived with would have been lessened.

I thought if my mom would just make up her mind not to act the way she did, she could stop. Self-discipline was what she needed to learn. Little did I know she couldn't because of the neurotransmitters in the brain that were not working properly. When this happens, it disrupts a person's thinking, feelings, mood, ability to relate to others and daily functioning. They can also have thoughts that others are cheating or plotting harm against them.

Teens tend to have the world revolve around them and I was one. Recently I read a book called *Why Do They Act That Way?* by Dr. David Walsh. That helped me understand myself as a teen. I felt unloved, worthless, and thought no one cared, especially God.

I had heard about a great and powerful God at church, but when I prayed, I didn't see He cared. "God" would tell my mom to not comb her hair, not take her meds or eat only bread and drink only water. Sometimes she told us "God" told her not to talk to us. She also believed she was "God's" bride and that He was coming for her. She sat at the piano with the hymn book open to "The Bride of Christ" and I would angrily tell her she was not God's bride. I would mock her. I didn't handle very well the things "God" told her.

This is just a small handful of what our family dealt with each day when Mom was ill and remained at home. Of course it wasn't God who really said these things, but my mom really believed He did. So can you see how confusing this could be? I thought "God" was mean for letting my mom believe the voices in her head. My anger grew.

10
DESTRUCTION

The walls I had started to build back in fourth grade around myself were stacking up and were being sealed with fast-drying mortar. In sixth grade, more bricks were added to my wall. An eighth-grade boy put his hands under my dress on the bus as I walked down the aisle to my seat. He laughed as he grabbed me in a very inappropriate way. I was mortified. I was menstruating at the time.

The summer before I was going into the eighth grade, this same boy, who was in high school by that time, saw me at the local swimming pool. He came up behind me and forced me against the wall of the pool so I couldn't get away. He then put his hand in my suit bottom. No matter how hard I struggled and told him to stop, he would just laugh.

I was too ashamed to cry out for help. I looked up to see if the lifeguard could see what was happening. Part of me wanted him to see and kick this boy out of the pool. The other part of me was so ashamed that I prayed he didn't see. After what seemed like an eternity to me, in reality maybe 30 seconds, he finally let me go.

I hated this boy, but I feared him more. I told no one. This era of time was when sex was not talked about, at least not in any families I knew. I felt dirty and wondered what I had done to make him do that to me. I buried all of this deep within. Years later, it was through a friend of one of my daughters that this incident came to the surface. I realized then that I had been raped. A young girl was thrown into a ditch by some boys and they proceeded to molest this girl with their hands. This incident went to court and the boys were charged with rape.

I often wonder if my mom's illness plus this incident fed the rebellion of my teen years and some of my destructive behavior.

On a hot, summer afternoon I walked into town with some of my friends. We saw a little trailer behind a building. We laughed and dared each other to break into it. Smug looks smeared across our faces and we bragged about how easy it was as the four of us were standing in a person's home. I wondered if the guy was at work.

I was scared. I wanted to get out. One of the boys opened the fridge and started throwing the eggs out. The others joined him, yelling and laughing. It didn't take me long to join in and totally trash the place. I felt no remorse while I was doing it. In fact, I did not feel bad until we stopped and there was nothing more that we could trash.

I stood in the middle of the disaster and saw what we had done. I wanted to cry but couldn't in front of the boys. What had I done? Why did I do that? I wanted to get out of there fast. All my anger and frustration, that I never expressed but rather stuffed inside me, exploded in a destructive way. I hated what I had done. I stood there deeply ashamed of myself.

When I got home, I cried and had a great fear that the police would find out and show up at my parents' door. I avoided going down that street for the longest time. I did not know how I could explain what I had done. I had no answer at that time.

11
SNEAKING OUT

When I was 14, I came up with the great idea of sneaking out with one of my siblings. We had asked my dad if we could sleep outside on the hay wagon to watch the Fourth of July fireworks. With Dad's permission, we put our sleeping bags on the hay wagon in the back yard. When we thought everyone was asleep, we walked the half mile into town. I am not so sure what I thought I was going to see in town. In reality, we saw the fireworks a lot better lying on the wagon looking up into the night sky. Maybe it was the adventure of sneaking out. I didn't really have a plan.

"Hey, let's go over to the cannery where the fruits and vegetables are processed," I said to my brother. As we wandered between the buildings with wooden crates stacked up alongside them, I saw a cop car. Quickly, we ran behind the crates hoping the cop didn't see us, but he did. Shining his light on us, he commanded us to come out. I know my heart was racing, wondering what Dad would say.

He asked, "Do your parents know where you are?"

We replied shyly, "No".

He put us in the back seat of the police car and took us home. I knew we were in trouble and the belt was coming our way!

The policeman knocked on the door. My dad stood there listening to the cop explain where he found us. Dad told him he would take care of it and thanked the officer for bringing us home. Dad didn't say a lot, which put more fear in me. He took his belt and whooped us on our rears. I never thought of Dad's discipline as abuse, just consequences to being disobedient. I had been disrespectful to my dad. He had trusted me.

Because of this incident with the police, rumors started spreading about me in town and in church. I was on the patio, petting the dog, when my dad came up to me and asked if I was having sex with boys. I looked at him in shock and disbelief and asked him where he had heard that. I had not even kissed a boy. I replied angrily, "No!" My dad said he believed me and walked away.

I confided in my best friend about what my dad had asked me. Timidly, she told me that the rumor had come from her mom. My friend proceeded to tell me that the rumor she had heard from her mom was that I had been caught having sex with a boy behind the cannery. I explained to my friend the real story of that night. I was deeply hurt by the rumor. Another brick added. I wondered if my dad had told some people about what my brother and I had done on the Fourth of July and it got distorted as others passed it on.

Do I believe the principalities of this world set out to destroy us? Yes! I look back at my life and see how the enemy used many circumstances to make me feel like I was worthless, to the point where I didn't care anymore. I wasn't strong enough at this point in my life to see through Satan's lies.

One night, when I was in bed as a young teen, I wondered if a man would ever want to marry me. Who would want me, if he knew about my mom? He would run. I was sure of it. I felt like my mom was ruining my life. I thought I was already tarnished because of that eighth-grade boy. The only man I could get would be in a graveyard. A corpse was all that would want me and was all I deserved to have for a husband, a dead man. I saw myself unworthy to be loved.

My rebellion and anger grew along with a disrespect for my mom. It spilled out even when she was well. I would tell her she was crazy. My mom didn't discipline me, but deep down inside it's what I wanted her to do. I did what I wanted, went where I wanted, unless Dad was around. I respected him but did a lot behind his back. There were times I did get caught.

Would it have made a difference if someone would have come into my life and mentored me at this impressionable time? Would I have listened? At that point in my life, I wanted to be a virgin when I married and I thought teens who smoked pot were stupid.

My aunt and uncle took me to a Christian conference. My dad wanted me to go, but my mom did not. When she was ill, she was always afraid my aunts were trying to take us kids away from her. I remember learning about God and feeling loved, sitting next to my aunt. On the ride home from Seattle, I was really tired and my aunt asked me if I wanted to put my head in her lap. I did. She ran her fingers through my hair and it felt wonderful. I felt so loved! I cried silently on her lap then fell asleep. I wished they had lived closer to me.

Like the bathing suit incident, the feeling was short-lived. I had to go home to my mom who was once again mentally ill and it was chaotic at home. This was a reality for me. The circumstances of life had once again stolen the joy I had gotten that one weekend.

Elaine Oostra

12

THE 70's

The 70's marked the last decade of the hippie era. 'Pot' was available pretty much everywhere for free. Teens were growing it in their parents' fields without them knowing. Parents were told to let their kids make their own choices. "Just be Free," was the big phrase. I was a prime target for the lies of the world at the age of 15 and set my life in a bad direction. I didn't care anymore about myself or life. I met others who felt the same way. I was mad at God for not healing my mom and I was going to show Him I didn't care about me just as I felt He didn't care. But I never doubted His existence.

Because of this attitude, I did some stupid things that were dangerous. Just outside of town was a train bridge. We would hang out there with friends and wait for the train. We would dare each other to either sit under the bridge or on the top, oil-soaked beams, or even on one of the wooden beams beside the track as the train would go by. The only place I dared to sit was under the bridge on the big rocks with the fast, roaring river only feet away and the train screaming overhead. I was never so scared in my life!

That summer I crossed over to doing many things that I had said and thought I would never do. I put myself in some awkward situations with boys. They thought they could do more with me than I wanted and then would tell me I was asking for it.

During this summer, I turned 15 and received my first kiss. It was awful! This boy was a friend of my older brother, and he asked me to go for a walk with him on a path that led to the river. I was young, naïve, and stupid. As we were walking, he pulled me to himself and started kissing me and more. I thought he was going to rape me. I pushed him away from me as hard as I could and slapped him. Then I ran as fast as I could. *What is it about me that makes boys think they can do stuff like that to me?* I, again, felt so dirty and ashamed. Because my relationship with my mom was so strained, I could not talk to her. It was out of the question.

Friends can make a difference in a teen's life. I wish I could say that my friends made a difference for the better, but they did not. Struggling teens seem to attract other teens who are struggling in life. My new friend, that I met while picking berries, talked smoothly and convinced me to go ahead and smoke some weed. I chose to do it. I knew it was wrong and I was even afraid of it, but there was just something enticing about it. It seemed that everyone was doing it.

My first introduction to 'pot smoking' was a couple of summers before. I was with my two cousins from another state. They were smoking pot with a boy in the car at the berry field where we were picking. I was sitting in the back seat while they were all smoking in the front seat. They told me not to tell. So when these new friends talked to me about smoking it, I figured I was old enough now and, besides, my cousins were doing it.

I went through that summer with my virginity still intact. I know God had protected me in spite of my stupidity. I put myself in a bad situation again in the middle of the city park. A boy I had just met pushed me to the ground and threatened to rape me right there. There was a man mowing the grass and I cried out for help as he drove by on the riding lawn mower. I thought he was coming to help me, but he said to me, "You asked for it." I felt so degraded. The boy left, angry. Again, it was confirmed that I saw myself as worthless.

I was clueless that my behaviors and how I dressed were sending signals. I was getting a reputation for doing things that I wasn't doing yet. The 70's were a time of very short dresses, halter tops, and short shorts. When my own daughters saw a picture of me as a teen, they asked me why I didn't have pants on.

My new group of friends in town came from families with alcoholism and other issues. I never talked about my mom. I felt comfortable with them yet, at the same time, uncomfortable.

I had been sheltered, in some ways, by going to a private school in another town and didn't know a lot of the "world's ways". I was never sure where I fit in. My friends in town would call me "goody two-shoes" because I went to a private school and not the public school most kids in my town attended. I wanted to show them I wasn't a goody two-shoes, so when they offered me a beer, I took it. It was awful and I never acquired a taste for it.

I met a guy one day with my new friends. He lived in an apartment in town. I didn't even know how old he was. He was part of the druggy group. He had brass knuckles and drug paraphernalia in his car.

"Dad this guy wants to take me out. Can I go?" I looked at my dad with the phone receiver in my hand. *Dad, please ask me about him. Say no!* I thought to myself.

My dad said, "Sure, go ahead." He didn't ask anything about him or where we were going. *Dad, don't you care?* I thought. I went to the party with the guy but hung out with my new friends that were there. The black strobe lights, mixed with pot smoking and drinking, filled the house. I don't think my dad had a clue what I was doing. I was mad he didn't ask. I wanted him to care.

My dad and I have talked about all of this. He told me he fell for the new parenting ways of the 70's and he regretted it. I forgave him long ago; I love my dad too much to be angry with him. My mom was clueless to everything that was going on. She was my mom, but that was as far as our relationship went. Loving her meant pain. She had left us so many times so I kept my distance, especially with my heart.

I don't know if our parents back then really understood what had entered our world as teens. Drugs were always around. We were protected for a time from the drug world, but it had reached our small towns and even the private Christian school I attended. What had been hidden before was now out in the open; drinking, drugs, the free sexual revolution and much more surrounded us. All you had to do was attend a rock concert and you saw it all.

Some parents learned fast, including my dad. Not only did my dad have to deal with living with a wife with mental illness but now with teen kids who were rebelling. In a sense, it was a different world than when my parents had grown up.

I watch my teen granddaughters now deal with things I never had to deal with. They have media at the touch of the finger with all the temptations coming at you whether you want it or not. When I was a teen, married couples on TV shows slept in separate beds. In my grandkids' world, non-married people lie naked in bed together and more, leaving nothing to the imagination on TV.

13
MENTAL HOSPITALS CLOSED

"What are we going to do with Mom? How will we live with her like that?"

When I heard the devastating news of the mental hospital being shut down, I felt sheer panic, anxiety, and anger at the same time. I wondered who we could blame.

I looked at my dad with fear-filled eyes. I wanted to lash out at someone, something! Who would watch Mom when we were at school and Dad was outside working? What if she...? Thoughts raced through my head of all I knew Mom could do. The voice commands in her head were real to her.

What if she went down to the river or walked down the road with her bizarre thoughts? She could not be left alone. This was for her own safety and maybe ours. There were times we couldn't find her and the police had to search for her. I always knew the faster our mother went to the hospital, the faster she got better. Now my fear was how would she get better? She didn't think she was sick! She would tell us we were sick and refuse to take her medication.

As I wrote about in Chapter 5, from the 1900's to the 1960's, people were put into mental hospitals for any small reason. Some were life sentences that may have had nothing to do with mental illness. Mental hospitals got a bad reputation and rightly so in some cases. People suffered from various forms of brain dysfunction, which was not as well understood when the policy of deinstitutionalization got underway.

From 1973-1976 the mental hospitals were shut down. Those on this commission should have spent time with families like ours before they made this decision. Did they ever live with a mentally ill person? I think they would have seen things differently. They would have seen the need for a very *restrictive setting*. It would benefit the ill person and their family in regards to safety.

The stress put on a family member to make the mentally ill person take their meds is beyond what I can explain. My dad tried in so many different ways to get our mom to take her medication including sneaking it in her food or drink, but she knew somehow, even though he never did it in front of her. I would be angry at my mom for not taking her medication and would leave the room, frustrated. It was usually not a pretty scene.

Imagine having to deal with mental illness or any illness, without a degree of a doctor or psychiatrist. As a family, we were forced to treat our loved one's illness. We had to jump through more hoops than you could count to get any help.

Taking away mental institutions was a sinking ship, like the Titanic. Didn't they say the Titanic was unsinkable? Deinstitutionalization is a continual sinking ship, a ship the government thought would stay afloat. But the untreated mentally ill now have lives that are virtually devoid of dignity or integrity. The unmedicated mentally ill person now thinks he or she has control over their own world in which their minds live.

In the past, my brother, who has a mental illness, would not commit himself to a rehab center for the mentally ill where he would be well cared for. We could not make him go. He voiced he wanted to be in control of his own life. Yet he caused havoc wherever he went. However in his mind and world, he was fine. (My brother, now in his 60's, is in an apartment and has a case worker that makes sure he is taking his medication).

The *"least restrictive setting"* frequently turns out to be a cardboard box, an abandoned building, a park, under a bridge, a jail cell, or a terror-filled existence plagued by both real and imaginary enemies. Imagine believing you see spiders coming through your skin. It's very real to you, so much so that you dig holes in your skin on all parts of your body to get them out. Or you believe there are snakes in your stomach and it's the devil tormenting you, so you need to kill yourself to get rid of them. How is all of this to be handled in the *"least restrictive setting?"*

Deinstitutionalization did not work then and it surely does not work now. Instead of being cared for and protected from themselves or others, the mentally ill are now housed in jails, on the streets, or in our case, being cared for by already struggling and untrained families. The whole system is messed up and the last person served is the mentally ill person. They seldom keep taking medication; rather they self-medicate with alcohol or other drug substances. You may ask, "Why don't they take their medication?" My answer is that they really don't believe, in their minds, that they are sick! Drug substance abuse along with mental illness is like pouring gas on a fire; it exacerbates schizophrenia. I have seen this in my brother. He has never held a 9-5 job. Schizophrenia destroys the mind and makes mentally ill people unable to cope with everyday life. They are so out of touch with the real world and can become a danger to others at times. We hear it on the news more and more.

I personally know of a mentally ill son who killed his father and almost his mother and little sister. This family had been crying out for help. However, some states require evidence of imminent harm to oneself or others for an involuntary commitment. This ties the family members' hands to get help for those they love.

Why do we wait for a mentally ill person to become a danger to themselves, family, and their community? I don't understand this way of thinking. When we cried out for help, we were told our mom had to hurt herself or one of us. Talk about feeling stress and frustration! As a teen, I figured the system out and would purposely aggravate my mother so she would hit me. This got the ball rolling for my mom to be committed and get the help she needed. I really did not like being put in this position; it caused emotional scars inside of me that needed healing. No child should ever have to be put in a position to make their mom hurt them in order to get the help needed.

When I did the research on the closing of mental institutions, so many emotions and memories went through my mind. When mental hospitals closed, the local mental health clinics took on the responsibility of outpatient care. I wanted answers. I wanted an understanding of this illness.

When I was 23, I sat in a small room at the end of a hallway at one clinic. In it was a bare desk and three plastic chairs. It felt cold to me and uninviting. The nurse entered the room and sat behind the desk. "How can I help you?" she asked.

"I have some questions about my mom and..."

She abruptly got up and barked, "I can't help you! We are here to help your mother, not you!"

"But I just want to ask you about..." again I did not get to finish. She walked out of the room. I sat there wondering what had just transpired. *Why can't they help me deal with this?* I wanted to yell at this lady, "Help me, please!" It was very clear to me that I didn't matter. I remember leaving angry and more frustrated.

The books I have since read, to help me understand mental illness, have been very focused on what the mentally ill person went through. There was nothing about what family members suffered living with an unpredictable person almost every day.

Families were not listened to by health professionals. 'Patient confidentiality' was given inappropriately as a reason for this. Families were often the main support for people affected by mental illness and they had a right to be treated as 'partners in care'. They needed information about the illness and treatment provided, about training, and support to help themselves as well as the person who was ill.

This was not provided for us. There was no help for us, as family members, to deal with or understand why our mom was the way she was.

I have seen a few changes from 30-some years ago. I can now look up websites that have many organizations that will help family members. This is so much more than what there was 30-50 years ago. I am so thankful.

"'For I know the plans I have for you,' declares the Lord, 'plans to prosper you and not to harm you, plans to give you a hope and a future. Then you will call on me and come and pray to me, and I will listen to you. You will seek me and find me when you seek me with all your heart. I will be found by you,' declares the Lord." (Jeremiah 29:11-14a, New International Version)

Schizophrenia is a chronic and severe brain disorder that affects approximately 1% of both men and women worldwide, as it has throughout recorded history. My mom had a lot of these symptoms.

Diagnostic criteria for schizophrenia (USA criteria; schizophrenia.com)

1. Delusions – false beliefs strongly held, in spite of invalidating evidence, is a symptom of mental illness

a. Paranoid delusions, or delusions of persecution: for example, believing that people are "out to get you" or the thought that people are doing things when there is no external evidence that such things are taking place.

b. Delusions of reference – when things in the environment seem to be directly related to you even though they are not. For example, it may seem as if people are talking about you or special personal messages are being communicated to you through the TV, radio, or other media.

c. Somatic Delusions are false beliefs about your body – for example, that a terrible physical illness exists or that something foreign is inside or passing through your body.

    d. Delusions of grandeur – for example, when you believe that you are very special or have special powers or abilities. An example of grandiose delusions is thinking you are a famous rock star.

    2. Hallucinations – Hallucinations can take a number of different forms. They can be:

    a. Visual (seeing things that are not there or that other people cannot see)

    b. Auditory (hearing voices that other people can't hear)

    c. Tactile (feeling things that other people don't feel or something touching your skin that isn't there)

    d. Olfactory (smelling things that other people cannot smell, or not smelling the same thing that other people do smell)

    e. Gustatory experiences (tasting things that aren't there)

    3. Disorganized speech (e.g. frequent derailment or incoherence) – this is also called "word salad"

    4. Grossly disorganized or catatonic behavior (An abnormal condition variously characterized by stupor/inactivity, mania, and either rigidity or extreme flexibility of the limbs).

    5. Negative symptoms - these are the lack of important abilities. Some of these include:

    a. Lack of emotion- the inability to enjoy activities as much as before.

    b. Low energy – the person sits around and sleeps much more than normal

    c. Lack of interest in life, low motivation

    d. Affective flattening – a blank, blunted facial expression or less lively facial movement or physical movements.

    e. Alogia (difficulty or inability to speak)

    f. Inappropriate social skills or lack of interest or ability to socialize with other people.

    g. Inability to make friends or keep friends, or not caring to have friends.

    h. Social isolation – person spends most of the day alone or only with close family.

Cognitive Symptoms of Schizophrenia
1. disorganized thinking
2. slow thinking
3. difficulty thinking
4. poor concentration
5. poor memory
6. difficulty expressing thoughts
7. difficulty integrating thoughts, feelings, and behavior

So I continue on with my story about how each of my memories, pleasant and unpleasant has shaped me and molded me into who God called me to be.

14
SWEET SIXTEEN

I was standing in the bathroom, combing my long blond hair, looking at myself in the mirror. I had just turned 16 that summer. *Kenny thinks I'm pretty. Am I?* The bathroom door was open when my mom walked by. "You are not that pretty, you know," she stated boldly.

"I know," I said, but to myself I thought, *Kenny thinks I am.* My mom grew up with the mindset that if you said anything to your children about them being pretty, you taught them to be vain. I found this out years later when sitting at lunch with my grandmother.

My daughter, who was 16 met us at a restaurant. When I saw her I said, "You look so pretty today!"

My grandmother scolded me. "Ach, you don't tell your children they are pretty. They might get a big head!" she said in her Dutch accent.

I smiled at my grandmother and told her I loved complimenting my girls. I loved my grandmother and I knew, that day, God had given me an understanding of why my mom made that statement to me so many years ago. My mom was also ill at that time.

I met Ken for the first time at my friend's house; her brother had just gotten home from the Army. I was only 15 at the time. I thought he was so handsome. He noticed me too! My freshman year, my friend would talk about the girls Ken was dating and I would feel jealous. It felt weird. He was older than me. I was wondering why I was feeling that way. It would be a year later before I would see him again.

I was dating a boy named Stan from Seattle who would come up to the bay, on the weekend, where we hung out and partied. My older brother had this big, old van that a bunch of us would drive out to the bay. We would open the back doors of the van and sit with our feet hanging free while my brother drove the bay strip, until the cops would pull us over and tell us to get into the van. We would meet other teens and hang out with them.

Stan invited us to a party that night with a bunch of his friends. I never really drank, just smoked pot. I wondered what it would be like to get drunk. I don't even know where the wine came from. I just remember lying on the beach with this boy and sharing a bottle of wine. I drank to the point I didn't taste it anymore.

The next thing I remember is lying in his car with my brother and some others, my head hanging out the window, repeatedly throwing up all over the side of the car. Stan took me to a friend's house and his mom tried to help me. There was talk of taking me to the hospital. I was so out of it. My brother took me home and carried me into the house where I continued to have the dry heaves.

The next morning I had to pick berries. All I could do was lay between the strawberry rows; my head hurt so badly! I never drank to that extent again. I don't understand people who brag about it at all.

Stan and I continued to date in spite of me messing up his car.

At the end of that summer, my friend and I were at the bay

and I saw Stan with another girl. I was devastated. A week before, he had asked me for his ring back. He had given it to me when I went to Seattle to see him at his parents' house for a weekend. He gave me the excuse that he needed it back because his mom didn't want him to give his ring to anyone. Believing him, I gave it back. I was so thankful I never gave myself fully to him. I had been tempted and came close to giving in to him.

"Let's go to your house. I want to get out of here." I said to my friend. I was mad. I had my parents' old white Ford car that you had to pump the brakes to get the car to stop. She lived about four miles from the bay.

When we got to her house I saw that her brother, Ken, was there standing outside. I was on the rebound and flirtatious. There were times my shy self was taken over by a bold personality. Most times I was very shy.

"You want to go for a drive so we can check out those brakes?" Ken asked me.

"Sure," I said sounding overly confident, still thinking of seeing my ex-boyfriend with another girl.

At an intersection, Ken reached over to me and kissed me for the first time. "Will you go out with me?" he asked. I hesitated realizing he was six years older than I was.

"Um, I am going to have to ask my dad."

"I would like to take you to the fair," he said. My over-confident attitude was leaving quickly and my shyness was right there to take its place. I really wanted to go.

"OK, I will ask. Call me tomorrow."

I really liked him; he was so handsome. But Mom was not doing well at all. *What if she scares him off? I can't have him come and pick me up at my house for a date! If he finds out about my mom, he won't want to date me.* All of these thoughts ran through my head as I was thinking about how I could have him avoid meeting my mom. *Why did I tell him I would go?*

I got off the bus that hot Friday afternoon in September. I had just started my sophomore year at the age of 16. Ken was picking me up in a few hours. I walked up to the house. *Mom is really bad right now. How am I going to handle this?* "Mom, Dad, is anyone here?" Everything was quiet.

I saw a note laying on the counter. "Kids, I took Mom to the hospital. Be back soon." I stood there, staring at the note. I hated that place and what it meant. I hated that my mom had to go there. At the same time, I hated what I had to come home to after school. What would she be like, manic or depressed? The depressed was easier to handle; she would just sleep. The manic was just that, manic! I wanted to cry, but I shoved the emotions down angrily.

Kenny was coming to pick me up; I didn't have to worry about him seeing my mom. That was a huge relief, but all my emotions felt like a tangled mess. I was so nervous about my date; I think I changed my clothes a couple of times. It was hot but I knew the evening would cool down. I ended up wearing a halter top and jeans.

Thank goodness Ken had his big army coat in the car because I did get cold. We had a fun time. Ken bought me a little cashmere sweater at the country fair. It was white with light blue and pink, wide strips. I still have it. I never knew why he asked me out again, but he did. I don't think I said but maybe two words on our first date.

During our dating time, I was still smoking pot until Kenny told me he wouldn't go out with me anymore if I continued. So I quit. I really didn't like how it made me feel anyway. I had some bad trips that really scared me. It wouldn't surprise me if it was laced with something stronger. I always got it free. I still smoked cigarettes and when we went to parties, I drank hard drinks. It helped me not feel so shy and made me feel more free to talk with his friends that we usually hung out with at the parties.

Ken and I were at a party at a local grange. The noise of the band came through the walls of the bathroom where I was hiding. *I don't know these people and they are all older than I am. What do I say to them?*

"Elaine, hey come out and join us," the girls outside the bathroom called out.

"She is really shy," I heard Ken say to them as he told them to coax me out. *Oh man, now it's going to be even more embarrassing to come out.* I knew that I couldn't stay in there forever. I eventually did come out.

I had a hard drink and that made me feel more at ease. Some guy pulled me out onto the dance floor; I was feeling pretty good until he asked me to go out to his truck. I said, "No way," and went to find Kenny. In a matter of five minutes, I had gone from overly shy to overly bold. I realize now that I came across as easy and guys got the wrong idea. I craved the attention, as wrong as it was, but I felt noticed. I was needy.

It is sad that I thought I needed alcohol or drugs to make me less shy which let me talk more easily with others. It's a false sense of security that allowed me to let my guard down. I am thankful now that God put a halt to the lifestyle that I was living as a rebellious teen. God knows me better than I know myself and loves me more than I had ever imagined. Sometimes His disciplines seem harsh, but in reality, it's His love for us that lets us suffer the consequences of our actions.

Elaine Oostra

15

PREGNANT

Rumors were flying around school about me being pregnant. I was wearing smock shirts as they were in style. Because I was dating an "older" boy, some classmates assumed I was messing around. I was doing nothing at that time to be able to get pregnant.

As Ken and I dated more, I thought, *Everyone thinks I "do it" anyway so we may as well go ahead and do it.* The standard I had set for myself long ago was crumbling around me. All the things I said I would never do, I had done. We talked about me getting on the pill, but I felt that meant I was doing something I should not be doing. I cried out for God to forgive me, but I didn't change anything.

It didn't take long for me to realize I was pregnant. This time, the rumors flying around the school were true.

I was running into the bathroom on the way to chapel to throw up. On my way out, a male teacher was standing at the entrance of the bathroom waiting for me. "Are you skipping chapel?" he asked.

"No," I said, "I was just going to the bathroom." I couldn't tell him the truth.

"Come with me," he said. He made me sit with him in the back row in the chapel with all the other teachers. I was humiliated.

The next thing I knew, the counselor called me into his office and asked me straight out if the rumors were true. I said, "Yes, they are." I couldn't hide it.

Reality hit me. There I was, 16 and a half years old and pregnant. At first, I was excited, until I was getting sick to my stomach all the time. I even had to ask the bus driver to stop alongside the road so that I could throw up. I stopped doing anything that would hurt the baby.

I told my dad I needed to go to the doctor because my lungs hurt when I breathed. My dad had asthma, so maybe he was worried that I might have it too. It was a great excuse and it worked. There was no way I could say, "Hey Dad, I think I might be pregnant. Is it OK if I go to the doctor?"

I situated myself on the short table with my knees in the air and my feet in stirrups. The doctor had made me put on a paper robe that tied in the back. I felt so embarrassed! This doctor had been our family doctor forever. He delivered all four of my mom's babies. While the doctor was examining me, he asked, "Elaine, are you dating anyone?"

I said, "Yes." He then confirmed my fear. I was pregnant. He asked if my boyfriend knew.

"Does he plan on marrying you?" the doctor asked me.

"Yes, I think so," I answered.

Later, Ken and I were sitting in the car after our date, when I confirmed to him that I was pregnant. "Will you marry me?" he asked.

"No, I think I might get an abortion or maybe give the baby up for adoption," I said with my head in my hands crying, knowing full well I couldn't do either. I was just desperate.

"No, you will not. You let me have the baby and I will raise it!" he firmly told me. "Please marry me," he said again.

This time I said, "OK, But don't smoke around me. It makes me sick to my stomach."

Ken took on the responsibility of asking my dad if he could marry me and telling him I was pregnant. He went to the barn while my dad was milking. I told my mom, who was doing well at this time. I was curled up on the floor in the front room. "Mom, I am pregnant," I said without looking up.

"Oh," she said. "What are you going to do?" I told her Ken was in the barn telling dad. "When are you getting married?" Mom asked.

"Soon, I think; you need to help me plan a wedding," I told her. Nothing more was said. I was glad.

Years later, I asked my mom what she really thought that day when I told her I was pregnant. She told me Ken should have known better. I smiled, "It takes two to make a baby. I was just as much at fault, Mom."

I quit school a little more than halfway through my sophomore year. I was embarrassed about my condition. Two years after I quit, another girl in my class became pregnant. She was the first girl in our Christian school to stay in school and finish her education. I was just too embarrassed to try and stay. I didn't even feel it was an option for me. I did get my GED when I was 40! I wanted to finish school. My kids gave me a graduation party!

Elaine Oostra

16
MARRIED

Less than a year after we met, we were married in my parents' front room, with just Ken's and my family and my best friend playing the piano. I was 17 and Ken was 22. Getting married in the church was not an option. I didn't care, I didn't want to. I was five months pregnant and felt I didn't deserve to be married in the church. My mom was doing well and organized everything for my wedding. I was clueless.

I had bought a white prom dress for $25 as my wedding gown. I think my veil cost more. In the bridal shop, I saw a pretty hair clip. I didn't have any money so I just took it and stashed it in my purse. I don't think Ken really had a clue as to the immature, needy girl he was marrying. I needed a maternity top too, so when shopping at another store, I stole one. Years later, God brought great conviction to me about this. Some sins just go hand in hand with other sins. My conscience was being seared.

We had a large reception in the church I had attended since I was born. It was a fun evening with some of Ken's friends putting on skits and his neighbor lady played her accordion. After the wedding, we went on a honeymoon to California. I had never been out of the state of Washington.

My marriage started with me seeking **my** happiness. I didn't know I was supposed to be seeking holiness. I was self-centered, not God-centered. I was going to do things my way. I didn't like God's way. He was distant to me and I felt He was uncaring.

We were two people with a ton of baggage standing before the pastor June 8, 1973. I had my bags packed and my ticket in hand, out of one life and into a new one. Prince Charming on the white horse had come to take me away! He was my very handsome hero. The only problem with this situation was I had taken all my issues with me, all my insecurities, fears, and frustrations that had deep roots in me. It took a long time to discover that my husband couldn't fill the emptiness in me, even if he would have been the perfect husband. No one on this earth could.

I didn't understand why I blamed him for all of our problems in our marriage. In reality, it was what I was trying to get from him that was the problem. I was trying to get from my husband what I thought I needed, craved, wanted, and desired: my value and my worth. I wanted to be rescued from my present life. I wanted to be loved. Did you know a man will run from a woman who insists he should complete her? He will tune her out. Men are not drawn to hysterical, needy women. They run and we chase. This drives men into their man caves, or they just leave, or lash out in anger.

What if it's a husband who comes into a marriage with his expectations of what his wife is to do? Could this be why there is so much divorce? Could this explain why there are so many murders?

I had rebelled greatly against God because of my mother's mental illness. This rebellion along with my unforgiveness greatly affected who I was as a wife and a mother.

I was an angry, bitter woman. I had hate in my heart. I was so angry at God for what I felt was a raw deal. As I write, I think,

Wow, I was fun to live with! Did everyone I know see this side of me? No, but then again, maybe. I felt I had to appear perfect to others. However, people who internalize eventually explode.

When you grow up with things out of your control, there is a tendency to want to BE in control. For some, things out of their control may have included substance abuse in the home, death, emotionally or physically abusive parents, etc. Being in control for me meant that all had to look perfect. When growing up, I thought all the homes of others had perfect families. Of course, they weren't. If things were not perfect and in control in my home, I felt it made me look bad.

It's called Pride. The thing about pride is that it calls itself names like low self-esteem, but it's pride, nonetheless. It kept me focused on myself and my needs and I excused it. Low self-esteem is insecurity. It damages relationships and hurts people closest to us. It stops us from being what God created us to be. Life becomes about us, but I was learning that life wasn't about me.

Elaine Oostra

17
LOSS OF CHILDHOOD FRIEND

Two weeks before the birth of our daughter, I received some devastating news. My childhood friend since second grade had been killed. She had just returned home, after being gone for a year. Ken was at his parents' house when he heard the news. He came home to tell me but then went back to see his parents. *Why didn't he stay with me?* I was feeling like everything was stacked against me.

I turned on some of my favorite rock music really loud and stretched out on the floor. Something inside of me refused to feel. My seventeen-year-old mind couldn't deal with this. My walls of self-protection at that point were so high. My friend's death just added more bricks. Her death also added more anger at God for being so unfair.

Ken told me a passing car didn't see her while she was walking alongside a dark country road. The car hit her and threw her 30 feet down the road into the ditch. She had left a stalled vehicle after her cousin had told her to stay in it and wait as he left to get help.

We were supposed to meet later that week with another really close childhood friend. The three of us had grown up together and had gone to the same church and school. We rode the school bus together every school day. We would pick berries, ride our bikes to each other's houses, and had birthday parties and slumber parties together during the summer months.

The last year before she was killed, we had separated, each going our own way. She and I both had not made good choices in new friends. I chose not to go to the funeral home to view her body; I didn't want that memory. I regretted later not seeing her one more time. This friend had missed my wedding and now was going to miss my baby's birth. I just asked God, *"Why?"* Years later, I found out that this friend had talked with her mom about a relationship with Jesus the night before she died. I was so thankful!

18
BABY

The first two and a half months we were married, we lived in a small, basement apartment in town with a bathroom down the hallway that we shared with another tenant. Ken took the car to work. I stayed in the apartment with nothing to do except sleep. I started watching daytime TV, but I was so bored! My stomach was growing. Sometimes I would walk uptown to the grocery store. I really didn't like to go out in public. I was embarrassed.

At the end of that summer, we moved to a rental house in the country. Sometimes Ken would get a ride to work so that I could have the car and get groceries. One day after shopping, I was walking to my car when another car pulled in beside me. It was a boy from my high school class. *Stop staring at me!* My stomach was huge! I got into my car as fast as my body would let me. I was humiliated; I didn't want my classmates to see me like this. In the 70's, most girls who got pregnant and didn't marry left town until the baby was born, or secretly had abortions. Seeing a seventeen-year-old girl walking around pregnant was not a common sight then. Today, it's no big deal. Embarrassment is not always bad. It meant I still had a conscience, knowing right from wrong.

Four months after we were married, we had our first-born daughter. I called my mom to come over and help me give the baby her first bath. Mom had been doing well. I was feeling safe with her. Being a new mom, I saw I needed her help and I don't think she minded at all.

Our baby girl had her nights and days mixed up. She cried a lot at night. I wasn't sure what to do. I tried all of the advice everyone had given me, but nothing helped. She would throw up the contents of every bottle. The doctor didn't seem concerned. He said she was getting what she needed from the milk and would get rid of the rest. There was no talk of changing the formula. I never even thought of breastfeeding. I just dealt with it and cleaned up after each incident. This went on until she was off the bottle. Dealing with a colicky baby at a young age was very difficult. I was frustrated and clueless. I was too immature and patience was not a virtue I had. This was a time in my life I would like to do over for a chance of being a better mom to my firstborn.

It breaks my heart when I see young pregnant girls today. Like I was, they are clueless as to the reality of caring for another human being for the next 18 years. Many of these girls are from broken homes, hoping this baby will give them the love they never had. It saddens me hearing this from teens. I tell them babies can't give. They need and they take.

Young teen moms don't understand their world will revolve around the baby who dictates all their time. Teens' worlds revolve around themselves. It's a rare occasion that I've seen a young teen have supportive, healthy parents to help them raise their babies. It takes a servant's attitude and maturity, ready to give their time for another, and knowing it won't be easy. I didn't have a servant's heart at 17. I was self-centered, looking for my own happiness. I could not imagine me trying to raise a baby by myself. It was difficult for me even with Ken there to help when he could.

19
DIRTY DIAPERS AND DIRTY COWS

Life had settled into a routine. I did what I said I would never do. I married a farmer. It's a lot of hard work, seven days a week. Ken was working in construction when we married. When that job ended, he got a job at a plywood plant that he hated. It lasted six months. "What do you think about milking cows?" Ken asked. I was resting next to him in bed thinking, *We would be together more!* "I hate the job I am doing, walking back and forth, flipping sheets of plywood day after day, and it's a dead-end job. It will be a lot of work starting my own dairy, but it's what I know and what I want to do," he told me.

"I can help you!" I said excitedly.

We rented our own dairy a few miles from my parents. I promised Ken I would do everything to help him in this new adventure. Because my brothers worked in the barn and us girls in the house, I had no idea really of what I had just promised. I was young and naive.

Every day, morning and night, I was in the barn with dirty

cows. I hated it! My job was to get the cows in from the field while Ken got the 40-cow stanchion barn ready for milking. I think we milked about 60 or more cows then. I washed the cows' teats ahead of Ken, who then put the milk machines on them. I had never done this before and was scared of cows.

Sometimes, when we had a cow or a new fresh heifer that kicked, it was my job to stand behind them and hold the tail at the base and press it towards the cow's back. This was not an easy task. It took a lot of arm power! This prevented the cow from kicking Ken when he put the milk machine on. I got peed on and pooped on more times than I can count. When the cow would cough with its tail forced up, I would get splattered everywhere with manure, even in my mouth!

Another job that needed to be done each day was to pitch the silage from the silo down a shoot. Then with a pitch fork, I put it into a wheelbarrow and pushed it out to the feeding trough to feed the cows, one wheelbarrow full at a time. This could be anywhere from 10 to 15 loads of this smelly silage.

Because we didn't have automatic feeders, we bucket fed the cows grain while they were being milked. This meant we had to fill the large buckets up with grain and dump the right amount in front of each cow. After milking, the manure needed to be scraped off the cement slab into the gutters. Then we would take the wheelbarrow again and scoop the poop from the gutters into the wheelbarrow and push it out to the manure pile outside the barn. Ken did all the milking and tractor work, field work, and much more, while I did a lot of the manual work. I refused to learn to drive the tractor.

I was thin and fit from all I did! Our daughter would sometimes be in the playpen playing in front of the cows and sometimes she got to go with my parents, who lived two miles away. This was farming life for most husbands and wives.

So there I was, 17 years old with a husband, cows, a colicky baby, and changing dirty diapers. My friends were going to prom, soon graduating, and some heading off to college.

Instead, I had to be in the barn with cow #33 that I hated and she hated me! This cow would claim every calf that was born. Ken would take a shovel out to the field to have as a weapon if she came after him when he was bringing in a new-born calf. I would head for the neighbor's barbed-wire fence that separated our fields and throw myself under the fence, to the other side. If I walked behind her in the barn or tried to wash her, she would kick at me. So, whenever I would feed her grain I would kick her head. Yes, it was stupid, but she would make me so mad.

I never really had any problem with other cows like I did her. One day, as I was wheeling the wheelbarrow out to the manure pile, #33 spotted me from the barnyard. I froze then quickly looked around for a place where I could run. I could see it in her eyes what she was going to do. The closest thing to me was about 20 feet away; it was the wooden hay bin feeder in front of me. Would I make it? I had no choice. She was coming at me fast! I ran and I dove into the trough feeder and crouched in the corner as far as I could. She tried to jump in and couldn't, so she started hitting the bin feeder with her head!

I was screaming and crying, all the while knowing with the milk pump on, Ken wouldn't hear me. I thought I was going to die there! Ken must have realized I hadn't come back into the barn. I heard him yelling at the cow and shooing her way. I got out, still crying and went back to work. No sympathy from Ken; there were cows to milk. This cow became meaner, to the point that we couldn't retrieve any calves that were born in the barnyard. She didn't care if you had a shovel. Off to the butcher she went. This was farm life. Ken was used to it, but I was not.

This was not my plan for my life. I went from one situation that I wanted to escape from to this. I resented it. I felt like life was always hard and against me. I had a lot of self-pity. I was no longer the center of Ken's world, work was. He married a little girl who had grown up with a lot of emotional baggage. Yes, he had lots of his own baggage too that he contributed. What a pair we were! Marriage was harder than I ever thought. Where did my prince on the white horse go? Who was supposed to rescue me?

Elaine Oostra

20
WHAT'S HAPPENING TO ME?

Reality set in; this was my life. I got depressed. I had no friends or social life except family. I was crawling back into a shell. There were no drinks at a party to rescue me and pull me out of my insecurity. I was intimidated by everything and my shyness that I already struggled with was becoming worse. Talking with others was hard. I wanted to hide.

One of my sisters-in-law took me over to her friend's house. I was really scared to meet new people. I had absolutely no self-confidence and I was afraid of my own voice. Sitting around the kitchen table, our hostess poured us coffee while we talked, only I didn't talk. I froze, looking at the coffee. Nervously, I picked up the cup with my hands shaking. I put it to my lips and tried to take a drink. I couldn't swallow and the coffee went down the wrong hole! I started coughing. Feeling embarrassed, I just wanted to leave and go home and hide.

What is wrong with me that I can't even drink coffee in front of someone I don't know? What is happening to me? I felt so worthless and unlovable. Being a mom and a wife was hard. Suicide thoughts entered my brain. No one knew. Fearful thoughts of becoming ill like my mom haunted me. These thoughts wouldn't go away.

Even though I didn't recognize it at this time in my life, God had His hand on me and had a plan for me. I was able to keep all of the feelings I had inside of me numb for a short time with alcohol, pot, and cigarettes. Being a mom, I had let go of those things. I came to full awareness and I had nothing to hide behind. God was slowly and patiently drawing me to Himself and making me face things I didn't want to face. It was all His perfect timing. This was not an overnight fix. This was going to be a process of years.

God doesn't have a watch or a calendar. He knew my prideful and stubborn heart, but it didn't stop the work He was going to do in me, and is still doing in me today. He is sovereign. He works all things out for His purpose and His plan.

The sovereignty of God is His total control of all things past, present, and future. He is always in control. All things are either caused by Him or allowed by Him for His own purpose and in accordance with His perfect will and timing. I really struggled with this, although I know now it was because I really did not know God nor did I understand Him. I also didn't trust Him and I wanted to be in control. None of this stopped what God was going to do in me.

"Yet for us there is one God, the Father, from whom are all things and for whom we exist, and one Lord, Jesus Christ, through whom are all things and through whom we exist." (I Corinthians 8:6, English Standard Version)

21
I HAVE TO LIVE !

I was pregnant again for the third time. I had had a miscarriage two months before. The doctor told me that nature would take care of the miscarriage, but something wasn't right. I never felt good. A few months later, I got pregnant again but had a lot of pain in my side that would make me double over at times. I had been in and out of the doctor's office, but he never could find anything wrong.

One night the pain was bad and my ears were ringing loudly in my head from the pain. Ken called my dad over to watch our daughter while he took me into the emergency room. By the time we got to the hospital, the pain had stopped. I had just been to my doctor in town that day and had a physical examination. He had told me that things looked good. He did, at one point, say it could be a tubal pregnancy, but I was not bleeding so he ruled it out. When at the hospital, they couldn't take x-rays because I was pregnant. They sent me home and told me to see my doctor again. I was 18 years old and scared.

My mom drove me to the doctor the next morning; the pain was unbearable for me. My mom waited outside in the car with my one-year-old baby. I slumped onto my side on the small bench in the waiting room, too weak to even sit up. *Why can't he find out what is wrong with me?* My name was called and I went into the exam room and reclined on the table with the blue robe on me once again. "Elaine," the doctor said as he pushed around my stomach, making me wince in pain, "I can't find anything wrong with you. Elaine, are you getting along with your husband?"

"Yes," I said, looking at him with a puzzled look.

"How about your daughter, is everything OK with being a mom?"

"Yes," I replied back. *Why is he asking me this?* I wasn't going to tell him how I really felt about being a mom. I knew what he would think.

"You know your mom...," he started then stopped. *I got it! He thinks I am sick like my mom! I knew it! He thinks I have mental illness, that I am imagining all of this pain.* I couldn't believe it. Being shy and easily intimidated, I dared not say anything to him. Instead, I stuffed my anger at him down inside of me. I got dressed, ready to cry. The pain was horrible and he didn't believe me. *Was I like my mom? Was I imagining this pain? It sure felt real.* I walked slowly, painfully out of the doctor's office and got into the car.

"Take me home, Mom." I just wanted to sleep. As we were going down the driveway, the pain worsened and something felt like it exploded inside me.

"Mom! I can't see!" I yelled out. I reached my hands out to feel around me and see if I could see them. I couldn't! My mom stopped the car in front of the house and I opened the door and stepped out. That was all I remembered. I awoke on the kitchen floor, my mom kneeling by me with a worried look. My daughter was standing there. *I have to live. She needs a mom!* My head hurt; I had cracked it open falling on the cement.

"What do I do?" my mom asked me. I told her to put my legs up on a chair. I thought it would help ease the pain.

"Call the doctor, Mom," I said in a whisper, strength draining from me. I listened as my mom calmly, yet fearfully, tried to convince the doctor to come. He asked her where I hurt. I told my mom to tell him, "Everywhere."

When he got there, he took my blood pressure and I saw fear enter his face. He had to make decisions quickly: who would take me to the hospital, who would take care of my baby, who would be in the office with the rest of his patients? I heard him discuss this with the office nurse on the phone. He knew now I wasn't crazy which relieved me. I knew I wasn't. He knew he had to take me, as time was running out. My mom stayed with the baby and was to tell Ken when he got home.

I was lying in the back seat of the doctor's car, numb, and wanting to sleep. I think shock had set in. I felt nothing. I kept hearing my name being called, "Elaine, don't sleep, stay awake!" I heard this over and over as I would drift off. Then I heard the doctor singing, "Glory, Hallelujah." He was calling out to God. I felt comfort. I had to fight! I wanted to live; I didn't want to die!

When we arrived at the hospital, the nurses quickly put me in a room and they cut my clothes off of me. I had been bleeding internally for some time now and had lost a lot of blood. I kept asking, "Can't I sleep?" Finally, they put the gas mask on me.

I awoke, asking if I could have more babies with one fallopian tube totally destroyed by the growing baby in the tube. Now I had lost two babies. They assured me that I could, but that it might take a while to get pregnant again.

Two months later I was back in the doctor's office confirming that I was pregnant again. Our second daughter was born, giving me a greater appreciation for life and for my babies. My search for God was beginning to grow. I knew something in my heart wasn't right and the void in me was growing.

22
THE VOID

We had all our parents and grandparents over after the baptism of our little girls. The tradition of the denomination we attended was to make a profession of our faith, which Ken and I did that same day we had our girls baptized.

My grandma came up to me and hugged me, "I am so happy for you!" she said to me. While her arms were still around me I thought, *But Grandma, something isn't right in me. I am a fake. I really don't have that faith the pastor talked about that we should have as parents to raise our girls, and I think if I die, I am going to hell.* I hugged my grandma back and thanked her for coming to the celebration. I knew about God. I knew He existed, but I didn't have a relationship with Him. He felt so distant from me. How could He love me when I was still angry at Him?

But God was tugging on my heart. It started by me noticing something was missing in my life and desiring that something. Having a husband, kids, and a home didn't fill that void in my life as I thought it would.

Nothing outwardly changed at this point. Life went on. But God was at work in me and around me, putting His plan for my salvation into place.

"'The wind blows where it wishes, and you hear its sound, but you do not know where it comes from or where it goes. So it is with everyone who is born of the Spirit.'" (John 3:8, ESV)

"even as he chose us in him before the foundation of the world, that we should be holy and blameless before him. In love he predestined us for adoption as sons through Jesus Christ, according to the purpose of his will." (Ephesians 1:4-5, ESV)

"For God so loved the world, that he gave his only Son, that whoever believes in him should not perish but have eternal life. For God did not send his Son into the world to condemn the world, but in order that the world might be saved through him. Whoever believes in him is not condemned, but whoever does not believe is condemned already, because he has not believed in the name of the only Son of God." (John 3:16-18, ESV)

I was the biggest condemner of myself. I thought God condemned me too. God knew all this, yet He loved me and wanted me to know of His love. He knew how to draw me to Himself.

I see all this now, years later, as clear as can be and I marvel at His work in me. But at that time in my life, I didn't see nor understand.

"just as the Father knows me and I know the Father; and I lay down my life for the sheep. And I have other sheep that are not of this fold. I must bring them also, and they will listen to my voice. So there will be one flock, one shepherd." (John 10:15-16, ESV)

23
SICK AGAIN

After about four years of being married, we bought our own dairy a fourth of a mile from Ken's parents' house. Ken put in a milking parlor. No more stanchion barn! We eventually hired someone to help with the milking and chores. My work in the barn lessened. We had another baby, a boy. We built a new house on the farm and let the hired man live in the old house.

One day, while I was out running errands, I decided to see my mom. I walked into the kitchen and took one look at her and knew. Her hair was not combed or curled, and was flat to her head. She had "that look" and wasn't dressed, but still in her bathrobe.

My heart sank and anger rose up in me and out of me. I started yelling at my mom. What I said, I don't remember. I think I yelled at her for not taking her medication. I was just mad and all the past and hard times poured out of me. What was our family in for again? The hospital was closed, so what was my dad going to do? Every time Mom got sick, I hoped and prayed it was the last time. Sometimes, not often, we would get a break for a few years.

"Not again!" I yelled out, "No, not again!" Anger rose up inside me. I said a word I never had said. "G__D___ you! I thought this was over!" I yelled at God and my mom. I was glad my kids were not with me. I felt like I had lost it. I regretted deeply using God's name in vain. I wondered if I looked and sounded crazier than my mom. I knew there was no way I would let my kids see their grandma like this. She could say off-the-wall things to them that may hurt them, like she did to me when she was sick.

A couple of weeks later, Dad and Mom drove to our farm and parked in front of the barn. Since my parents no longer milked cows, they would get their milk from our milk tank.

"Why won't Grandma come out of the car?" my kids asked. When my mom was well, she loved on her grandkids and would greet them warmly whenever she and Dad came over.

"She is sick and doesn't feel well," I told them. I was mad at my dad for bringing her over. I wanted to protect my kids from seeing what this illness looked like and what it could do. I didn't want to answer any questions my kids might have. I didn't have any answers for them as to why grandma had this illness. I avoided my mom as much as I could when she was ill. We lived about 20 miles from my parents so it made it easier and it was my excuse.

I continued to stuff the bitterness and the effects this disease had on my family, but it began to penetrate into my dreams at night. I was yelling at my mom in my dreams, physically angry with her. I felt out of control. Sometimes I felt or saw a demonic presence in my nightmares. I jolted up in bed and wondered if Ken had heard me scream. I was sweating and my heart pounded. This was a reoccurring nightmare. *God help me,* I cried in my heart. I was so ashamed of my dreams and how I had treated my mother. I never told anyone.

When we had been married nine years, we had our fourth baby, a girl. Life revolved around kids and the farm. Life and marriage had its ups and downs. My two oldest were old enough to go to Vacation Bible School, so I thought I would help and teach a class. I had never done anything like that before and was scared. I was reading the little kids a Bible story and an emotion I had never experienced before came over me. I felt like crying, but it felt wonderful at the same time.

What I didn't know was God was touching my hard heart with His Word that I had ignored. It's His Word that changes us. It's powerful and full of life. Two years after reading that Bible story, God called my name. I heard and answered.

Elaine Oostra

24

BORN AGAIN

My sister-in-law invited me to go with her to a Bible study on the Women of The Bible on Monday nights at our church. I found myself saying yes. I had grown up in the church, went to Sunday school, catechism, and a Christian school. I got it six days a week. I knew all of the stories of the Bible. I had memorized scripture. I thought I knew all there was to know, so I never opened a Bible. I had no desire to do so. I knew of God, but I didn't *know* Him. He existed to me like a distant relative I had heard of but had never personally met and didn't care to talk about.

I had an aunt that talked about Jesus all the time and it drove me nuts! I thought she was a fanatic. People I went to church with never talked like she did. It's kind of ironic; I went to church all my life, yet it was thought to be weird or fanatical to talk about the very reason why you went. We never talked about our faith. Something was different about my aunt; I was drawn to her at the same time that I was thinking that she was weird. At one point in my life, I found out that this aunt wanted to take me in whenever my mom was sick, but my grandfather wouldn't let her because she was of a different denomination than my grandfather. The difference in their doctrine was when to baptize. I would have loved to have stayed with my aunt.

Going to the Bible study with my sister-in-law put a deeper hunger in me for God's Word. When it was over, I felt unsatisfied. I wanted more. God was tugging on my heart even stronger and I didn't know it. I didn't understand why I was feeling the way that I did.

When I was 28, I was asked to attend a Bible study called Precepts. I heard it had a lot of homework. Again I don't know why I said yes, but I did. When I got my book, I thought, *Oh man, what did I get myself into?* There were five days of work each week! I hated homework. This felt like school. I did the work and went to the study. The study was on the Book of John. We had to look up Greek and Hebrew words and look up a ton of verses.

One day I was just mad at the study book and threw it across the floor and thought, *Why am I doing this? This is work!* I was getting nothing out of it. The Bible was boring. Had I not done enough by going to church, Sunday school, and Christian school all my school life? I looked at the book on the floor. *I paid twenty dollars for that book and I am going to finish it, even if it makes me work!* This is the "Dutch" in me; don't waste what you pay for.

I was standing at the end of the counter with my Bible study book. The kids were at school and my youngest was napping. I think we were in Chapter 3 of the Book of John. All of those years in church and nobody, that I remember, ever told me that I had to be born again. Maybe I didn't listen or didn't have the ears to hear. However, there it was in black and white in chapter 3 verse 7. You must be born again.

"Do not marvel that I said to you, 'You must be born again.'" (John 3:7, ESV)

"For God so loved the world that He gave His only Son that whoever believes in him should not perish but have eternal

life." (John 3:16, ESV)

Even though I memorized this, it didn't change my heart. It just stayed in my head and puffed me up with knowledge, but there was no heart change. I had never read it in this whole context. It hit me; God's Spirit blew on me! No, I didn't feel the wind; I felt love like never before. He breathed life into me. God loved worthless me! He loved me. The Holy Spirit came into me right there at the end of the counter while I was reading my Bible. I read and reread. I couldn't take it all in as the words came alive to me as never before. I could see and feel what Jesus was saying to worthless me! Just a few minutes ago they were just words on the page and were boring with no meaning to me. Now I wanted to go to my front door and open it up and yell out to the world that I was born again, loved by God! I was saved and I knew it! I never had that assurance before.

"who were born, not of blood nor the will of the flesh, nor the will of man <u>but of God</u>." (John 1:13, ESV)

"You did not choose me, <u>but I chose you and appointed you that you should go and bear fruit and that your fruit should abide,</u>" (John 15:16a, ESV)

God chose me and I had a purpose. I couldn't save myself. I didn't ask Jesus into my heart, He just came! He knew me before the creation of the earth. I devoured the Book of John.

That next Sunday I couldn't believe how good the pastor had gotten in his preaching from the last week. I was blind, but now I could see and hear. I was so excited about what he was preaching. It took everything in me not to stand up and shout, "Amen!"

The word "believe" took on a whole new meaning. I read that even the demons believed and shuddered. When I read about believing and being saved in God's Word, I learned that action always follows. I would have to bear fruit and show that I was His disciple. I could no longer be a pew sitter.

God gave me an unquenchable thirst for His Word when He saved me. People even noticed something different about me. Believing meant totally surrendering my life to Christ. It was no longer my life. It meant trusting God with everything and obeying Him even if I didn't understand His ways. God had a lot to teach me about trusting Him. This was not the end. Being saved was just the beginning. When God chose me, he appointed me to go and bear fruit. I had a new desire to be obedient to what God asked of me. I am so thankful for His patience in teaching me obedience. I am a slow learner.

I wrote my testimony for the church newsletter. I remember one person coming to me and telling me she really enjoyed what I had written and this started a new long-lasting friendship. I treasure this friendship. We have gone through a lot together. It's now going on almost 30 years. I had prayed for Christian friends; I didn't have any. God abundantly has continued to supply this need in me for Christian fellowship with other women. He knows our needs as women.

My desires also changed in things I used to do. Reading romance novels and watching soaps now seemed so pointless, a waste of time and meaningless. Being on the phone and gossiping about others left me feeling awful. So when that phone would ring and I knew who was calling with more juicy gossip, I didn't add to the conversation and would say I needed to go, "Good-bye." The phone calls to me stopped. My taste in music changed; I wanted music that glorified God. The secular music reminded me of details in my old life that I wanted to forget. I also thought before that my kids needed to be popular in school in order to make it in life. Now I just wanted them to know Jesus. I wanted everyone to know Jesus!

I overheard a conversation in which I was the main topic from some who knew the old me. "Elaine is taking this religious thing too far; she isn't going to be any fun anymore." I smiled and thanked God that my new faith was showing. Personally, I thought I was becoming way more fun.

But I was still a very quiet person. Now I was a shy, saved

person. I was scared to answer a question in Bible study, and hoped I wasn't asked to pray out loud. I also was attending another Bible study in the evening about marriage called "Strike the Original Match," by Chuck Swindoll.

I attended the study because I wanted a Godly marriage and I thought Kenny was the one who needed to change, so I was going to change him. When I got the book and read the first page, it said the one who does the study is the one who needs to change. What? I was mad again at a Bible study. I felt like I was the one always doing the changing. Ken was the one who needed to change and I was good at helping him out.

I laugh at myself now in thinking of how I would tape verses to the toilet seat knowing he would for sure see them there! One had to remove the paper to lift up the seat. He would even find verses in his lunch sack. The ones taped on the fridge I claimed were for me but secretly hoped he would read them. I was going to help God out, but in reality, all I did was fill myself with frustration over something of which I had no control.

All of my "issues", unbeknownst to me, had spilled into my marriage. I had a great need to be "in control". God had a lot of refining to do in me. I didn't trust God with Ken any more than I did with my mom. The two became tangled into one person in my mind.

All I succeeded in doing was alienating my husband. I fell into the great sin of self-righteousness and pride. There were pure motives in my heart too, but most were not. I really wanted Ken to believe like me so "my" life would be better and we could look like the perfect family that I thought others had.

Elaine Oostra

25
IMPATIENT

Ken was not changing fast enough for me. The root of bitterness and anger grew. Ken even told me one day that I never smiled anymore, that I was always walking around mad and if that was what a Christian was like, then he didn't want any part of it. That made me angry! Truth does sting.

I cried out to God to help me. The Lord softly replied back to me, *"Elaine, look at the paper. There is a line down the middle. I put you on one side of the line and Ken on the other. I will teach you, Elaine, who I want you to be, and I will teach Ken who I want him to be. Stop meddling in my business with your husband. Elaine, let go and entrust Ken into my care."* How I wish I could say I did exactly what the Lord told me that day. God had to remind me daily many times and still does.

God had a lot to change in me and I wanted to change. Our pastor's wife was leading the marriage study. She had a bubbly personality to which I was drawn. After the Bible study, she would have each one of us pray out loud. *Please don't ask me to pray out loud!* Fear rose up in me and my heart pounded as she looked around the room. A sigh left my lips when she asked someone next to me. Maybe she saw the fear on my face.

This fear bothered me about myself. I wanted God to use me, but how could He when I was so afraid that I would sound and look stupid. I was still very self-centered and only thought about me and *my* comfort place. I didn't know how to pray.

The enemy would have loved to have kept me incapable, insecure, and unusable. He had kept me there in the past without a fight. But the fight was on now! I learned, *"Greater is he that is in me than he that is in the world" (I John 4:4b, King James Version)!* The only way to get over the fear of praying out loud was to pray feeling afraid. I had to do whatever I needed to do, afraid. Christ was in me; He would give me the power and strength to do whatever there was to do no matter how inadequate I was.

I had to get over my old self; I was a new creation in Christ! Was I going to trust Christ or not? It was not about me anymore and what was comfortable to me. If Christ could hang on that cross after being beaten unrecognizably with nails driven into his hands and feet for the sins of the whole world, how can I say, "I am too shy to pray out loud?" Will God and I part ways here?

This may seem like such a small thing to some, but to me, it was a real fear. God wanted to grow me, to conquer my fears. He put this desire in me.

Later I found out a certain amount of fear is good; it keeps us relying on God and not self and keeps us humble. I really listened to others and how they prayed. It was like they were talking to a friend. They didn't use elegant words like I thought I had to do. The evening came when I was asked to close in prayer. Silently I prayed, *"God show me and teach me what you want me to say, I have no words."*

"Good," the Lord said, *"then I can speak through you."* The Lord spoke through me with my shaky, nervous voice.

26
TIPPED SCALES

Beware of the enemy and his tactics. He can try and make you ineffective as a believer. He deceived Eve in a perfect world. He can deceive us.

"Therefore we must pay much closer attention to what we have heard, lest we drift away from it." (Hebrews 2:1, ESV)

"Therefore, brothers, be all the more diligent to confirm your calling and election, for if you practice these qualities you will never fail." (II Peter 1:10, ESV)

The enemy saw my great need to be loved by those around me. I knew God loved me, but I had an idol. I wanted love with flesh on it. My idol was Ken. Earlier on when we were first married, we were walking away from the barn when Ken turned around and said to me, "You need to get me off that pedestal you put me on." I think the Holy Spirit spoke through him that day, because it never left my mind. God wanted to be my all in all. He wanted to teach me my deepest needs are only satisfied by Him alone. I had a lot to learn. A lot of my bitterroots were from not feeling loved by others and feeling rejection. I was still subconsciously looking for my approval from people more than from God.

I desired to obey God with every fiber of my being. I hadn't wanted this before. I wanted to love my mom. I wished to be a good daughter to her. I longed to be a good wife. I wanted all of these awful feelings in me to change. I became aware of everything that was not good in me.

Naively, I thought I could handle it when my mom got sick again because of this change in me. Did you notice the "I"? Right off the bat, I started running in my own strength, kind of like Peter in the Bible; I can relate to him. I had no idea all the areas in which God wanted me to grow and heal. God is so good. In His patience and love, He gently pried loose one brick at a time from my self-made wall. It's like He asked me to examine each brick and why I put it there. That way I could really look at it and let it go, because I have learned to trust Him in that area of my life. When I tried to tear the bricks down myself, I always seemed to make a mess and add on more bricks instead.

I wanted Ken to fulfill all my wants and needs. I wanted him to give me the love and affection that I felt I didn't get growing up. Now that I was a born again Christian, I for sure wasn't getting what I wanted from Ken. I talked to my pastor about this because the things Ken said to me really hurt.

Because of this conversation with my pastor, I wrote this story.

Sarah looked out her kitchen window, while washing her evening dishes. A tear slowly slid down her cheek. "Why God?" she questioned, "I thought when I became a Christian, life would get better. Why is my husband rejecting my new-found faith in You? God this hurts so badly!" Memories of yesterday floated in her mind. Sarah was doing her Bible study at the dining table when her husband came home from work.

"Is that all you have to do all day? If you have time to do that, you

have time to straighten out the checkbook," he yelled at her. Sarah had no idea how to do the bank statements and see if all the checks came through. No one had ever shown her. She didn't understand why he was so angry about her studying the Bible? She defended herself by saying she had just sat down.

Sarah had started to go to a Bible study a couple of months before. It made her feel alive; she was feeling a joy in her heart she had never felt before. Assurance, that's what it was. Jesus had died for her sins! "Personal" they called it, having Jesus as your personal Lord and Savior. She wanted to open the door of her house and yell it to the world that she was saved! She wanted so badly to share this news with her husband; she had tried in different ways only to be told she was a religious fanatic. "Oh Lord," she cried, "Why is he doing this to me?"

She kept her pain to herself. She saw what she thought were other happy couples in church. Were they able to share their faith with each other? Sarah's husband did come to church with her once in a while only because she nagged him. After all, he was the one who thought their two daughters should be baptized and that they should become members of their church. This is what totally confused Sarah. Why did her husband think membership and baptism were important, but not a personal relationship with the Lord? If you did talk about a relationship with Christ, you were crazy. "That's the way pastors talk. Do you want to become a pastor?" her husband would ask her.

Sarah and her husband were arguing a lot lately since she had been saved. She didn't want to do some of the things she used to do. She was being called a goody two-shoes and hearing things like "Who do you think you are? Miss Perfect? You should have married a minister or a missionary."

Sarah looked at her reflection in the kitchen window; tears were streaming down her face. She was glad the children were in bed and her husband was at a meeting for the evening. She went into the front room and knelt by the couch and folded her hands. "Lord," she prayed, "I am having a really hard time loving my husband. I am so angry with him. I do not understand his rejection of my faith in You. I do not understand why You would save me only to have my marriage get worse instead of better. I read about other couples becoming Christians together and sharing their faith with each other and going to Bible studies together. Lord, I confess I was so jealous when I read it and I wanted to throw the book in the garbage. Lord, I do not understand your ways. But Your Word says to trust in You, that You do things differently than we do. Lord, help me. I feel so alone. Is my faith in You crazy? I am starting to doubt You. Forgive me. I wonder if following You is worth it. It's rocked the boat and I like things smooth, Lord. Lord, make me strong in You and help me to again love my husband. Amen." Sarah went to bed early that evening. Her crying had given her a headache.

What Sarah didn't understand yet was that God was using this trial in her life to help her grow in her trust in Christ. God had heard her prayers on wanting to be all Christ wanted her to be. She had asked God to mold her and shape her into who He wanted her to be. She had asked God to refine her like gold. Gold must go through fire first, be boiled, and have all the yucky stuff scraped off. Then the gold is poured into its mold and polished. The finished product is shiny and beautiful.

"Sarah, I see your pain and hear your prayers. I know it hurts to be ridiculed for your faith. Don't give up. I am testing your faith to be genuine. I am with you, Sarah," the Lord said to her as she placed her head on the pillow.

Sarah awoke early the next morning, the sun streaming into the bedroom. It felt warm. Sarah rolled over facing her sleeping husband. "Lord, help me to love him today," she silently prayed. Sarah kissed him softly on his cheek. "Good morning, Honey." I have not done that in a long time, Sarah thought.

Sarah made an appointment with the pastor to meet with him that afternoon. She had to talk to someone about the confusion she was feeling about her faith and the conflict it caused in her marriage. She was afraid of crying in front of the pastor so she wrote out what she wanted to talk about.

"Hello, Sarah. How can I help you today?" Sarah nervously handed him the letter and explained her fears of crying. The pastor kindly took it and read it. After he finished reading it, he thought for a minute. "Sarah, do you remember what you were like before you really got to know Christ and what He had done for you?"

"I guess kind of like what my husband is like now," she replied. "I went to church because I had to, I never read my Bible, and I saw no need to read it. I would have never gone to Bible study. That would have been weird!"

"Sarah, when your husband sees you reading and studying your Bible, he is very much convicted because he knows he should be in God's Word too," the pastor said to her.

"Boy," Sarah replied, "I do remember feeling that way. I stayed away from "those" Christians for that very reason."

The pastor held up the replica of a scale with a bowl on each side that was sitting on his desk. He told her, "Before you were saved, you both were an even weight on the scale. But now the scale has tipped and feels off balance. Let's pray for God to balance the scale." The pastor and Sarah bowed their heads and prayed for her husband's heart and that their faith would grow and Sarah would be patient with God's timing.

"In this you rejoice, though now for a little while, if necessary, you have been grieved by various trials, so that the tested genuineness of your faith – more precious than gold that perishes though it is tested by fire-may be found to result in praise and glory and honor at the revelation of Jesus Christ. Though you have not seen him, you love him. Though you do not now see him, you believe in him and rejoice with joy that is inexpressible and filled with glory, obtaining the outcome of your faith, the salvation of your souls." (I Peter 1:6-9, ESV)

27
THE LIE THAT I NEED TO FIND MYSELF

When all my kids were in school, I started thinking about getting a job outside of the farm. We had a regular hired man, so I didn't need to be out there as much and our kids were doing barn chores. I thought I needed to "find myself." I soon realized that I took "myself'" with me wherever I went. Instead of finding myself, I realized I was searching for who God created me to be.

I didn't want to work on Tuesdays if I got a job. This was my Precept Bible Study day. I knew I needed it to encourage me and help me grow into the woman God called me to be. I loved learning the Bible.

Some of my friends had gotten jobs. The culture was really telling women they could do it all; they could be a mom and work. If you said you were a "stay-at-home mom", it felt like you were looked down upon. What I see now is that it was easier to go to work than to have to deal with raising kids which I felt was the hardest job on the whole earth! Then when your husband's business is out of the back door of the home, it adds to the work of being a mom and a wife. But God was going to use this experience to grow me more.

In our town, there was a cute Dutch bed and breakfast in a windmill with a gift shop under it. A lady that I went to Bible study with worked there. She told me of a job opening and asked if I would like to work in the hotel, cleaning the six rooms. I was 33 years old and on a new adventure; it was my first real paycheck job!

This new job was fun, even though it was cleaning. I was able to work with great women. The six rooms all had different Dutch themes, each one unique. We took great pride in making the rooms beautiful. After I had been cleaning for about four years, my friend, who worked with me, asked if I ever saw myself doing something different. Sitting in a hot tub bath I was cleaning I answered, "This is all I will ever be able to do. I didn't graduate from high school." I really believed that about myself. But God had other plans for me. He knew me and He was not going to let me put limits on myself. I was hiding in this job. It was safe.

Shortly after this conversation, my friend, Betty, asked me if I would be interested in working in the gift shop and taking the reservations for the hotel. I went to church with Betty. She saw something in me that I didn't see in myself. I stood there speechless. "Betty," I said, "I have never worked in a job like that. I don't know anything about cash registers. I won't know how to answer the phone right!" Fear filled me, yet, so did excitement and I heard myself tell her, "Yes!"

I went home and thought, *Why did I say that? I will make a fool out of myself. I can't do this! If Betty really knew me, she would regret asking me.* Confidence was something I did not have. *"God, if You want me to do this, please help me."*

I surprised myself as I caught on quickly to the things Betty taught me. We had to wear Dutch costumes; I had a Dutch dress and Dutch bloomers with wooden shoes. I found that I enjoyed talking with customers. We had tour buses that came through our Dutch town. People from other countries, especially those from Japan, loved to stand beside me in my Dutch outfit and have their pictures taken.

After working in the gift shop for about three years, one of the men from the head office came to me and asked me if I would like to be the manager of the shop. The manager, who was quitting, had highly recommended me. I was terrified! I was afraid of failing and wanted to stay in a safe place. I said no, even though I knew that place inside and out. When people called for reservations, they wanted to know which room to stay in and we had to describe each one. Cleaning the rooms for four years made me an expert and I loved describing the themes to the people. A new manager was hired. I trained her and we had fun working together. However, throughout the year, I saw I was doing a manager's job.

The new manager quit for another job offer. I went to the head office person and said I wanted the job. They were pleased. God was changing me. I was overcoming fears. I saw what I had to offer. I enjoyed people that I met from all over the world. I loved decorating the gift shop and making displays, which was a must in this job.

The owner complimented my work. It was fun going to gift shows and buying for the shop. The owner told me, "Treat this place as if it was your own, I don't want to be bothered with it." So, I did. I felt appreciated. This job was giving me something that I needed, but it consumed me. I was feeling frustrated at trying to keep everything up at home and then work. I had trained my family well in expecting me to do it all. I was trying to juggle everything. I was, at times, putting in long hours at my job. I also had hired my oldest daughter, who was in high school, to work part time at the gift shop. Our other kids were active in sports. At this same time, I was also taking a night class one night a week on Christian Lay Counseling.

The one thing that hit me hard in taking this nine-month class was when our teacher said to us, "You can help someone through counseling only as far as you yourself have been healed in your own hurts." I had seriously thought of becoming a counselor. I have noticed hurt people want to counsel others and not deal with their own deep-seated issues. That was me. I saw I had a place in my life that I was stuck, my relationship with my mom when she was ill.

God used this class to take the cap off the well I had kept sealed for the last few years in dealing with my mom. There were so many emotions buried deep inside. God knew in His sovereignty when it was time for me to deal with this.

I will never forget the incident. One evening, I walked over to the kitchen sink where my son, who was 11, was washing the dishes. I picked up a dish out of the drying rack. It was so full of grease. He had washed the frying pan first with grease in it. I lost it! I picked up a wine glass that he had washed and showed him how dirty it was still. Then I took the glass and threw it against the cupboard door. It shattered into a million pieces. I stood there, shocked at what I had just done. My son said, "Mom, I will do the dishes over. I will do better!" He was crying. I gently told him how sorry I was and told him that I would finish. I asked him to forgive me. I explained it wasn't his fault; it was me, not him.

I felt awful. *What is wrong with me? Why did I do that? "Oh dear God, please help me. I can't do this anymore. I can't keep doing everything. I am so tired."*

I thought back to the lay counseling class I took. "You can help someone through counseling only as far as you yourself have been healed in your own hurts." Pride was keeping me from asking for help. *What if getting counseling meant I was like my mom? What if Ken didn't think I needed it? What if he didn't want to pay for it? What if...?* All these questions went through my mind.

My heart pounded when I went to him to talk about it. I rehearsed in my mind what and how I was going to tell him. But my mind was made up. Even if he said no, I was going! "Ken, don't say anything until I am finished. I need to go see a counselor. I will pay for it with my own money. I am having a hard time and I don't know why. I am angry all the time." I explained to him.

"I don't know why you have to pay someone to talk to them," he said.

"I am going even if you don't want me to. I need to do this!" I said firmly and walked away.

I called the counseling center that I took the class with and set up an appointment. I was scared and nervous sitting in the waiting area. *What am I going to say? I don't know how to start. Maybe I could just cancel and go home.* I was struggling in my marriage, but I didn't want to talk about that. I am not sure why. Maybe I didn't want to admit that I was feeling like a failure as a mom and a wife.

My name was called. The counselor was really young. *How is she going to be able to help me?* When she asked me why I came, I said I needed to talk about my mom. I had no idea how entangled Ken and my mom had become in my mind.

Pain, when not dealt with gets transferred over to others.

Elaine Oostra

28
LETTER TO MY DAD AND MOM

I recently found this letter, dated December 22, 1989, when I was going through some of my parents' things. I wrote it before I went into counseling and the content surprised me. I'm pretty sure my mom was 'well' by how I felt about her at the time of writing the letter. When she was 'well', I would feel fine about her and stuff everything else inside. If she was sick, I distanced myself from her. These were not words I would have written if my mom was sick.

There was a war inside of me. My emotions were dictated by my circumstances. Yet, this is the first time I voiced to my parents how I felt about them. God knew the healing work He was going to do in me.

Dear Mom and Dad,

I just want to tell you I love you both very much. There is a lot I want to say to you. It's not easy to put into words. First of all, I am thankful to the Lord for putting me into your lives, that I am your child. Life was not always easy, but God never promised it would be. I know that it is the trials in our lives that mold us into the image of Christ. I don't look back and say, "Why, God?" I look back at our life as a family growing up and say, "I understand now." I feel blessed to have you as my parents! I see how much God loves me. He knew what it would take to make me turn to Him.

Dad, you are a great example to me. You taught me, by action, to stick it out in a marriage, no matter how tough things get. You made the statement once, "You are married and out of the house. You don't come back to live." Sometimes when Ken and I would have a fight, I would remember this and knew we had to work out our problems. It also made me turn to the Lord. Thank you, Dad, so very much! You now know how much this has helped me. I used to look back over my life and only see the bad times. But the Lord is replacing them and showing me all the good times. We didn't have much money, but that didn't matter. The hiking trips are special memories to me. You took time for us. Going to the dam, the state capital, and lots of hiking was an adventure!

Mom, you have been through so much in your life. I have only thought about me and how your illness affected my life. Forgive me. The Lord has been showing me a lot. Thank you for all the times you took care of my kids. Thank you for loving them and praying for them.

You are wonderful grandparents! It's funny that it's not until we have our own children that we can sympathize with our own parents. We stop passing judgment. Parenting is the hardest job in the world. So many times, I feel like giving up. Then I remember what we put you through. If you can do this, I can do this, but only with God's help and wisdom from Him. There is so much more I want to say, but I don't know how to put it into words.

Love, your daughter, Elaine. I love you both so much.

These are my reflections today of this letter. I thought I had arrived in my healing because I was saved! Yes, the finished work was done at the cross, but I still had to walk through it. I wanted microwave healing and God wanted crock pot healing in me. I did not fully understand yet ALL the work God wanted to do in me. He didn't use a wrecking ball on my wall. He took one brick out at a time. His grace and His mercy are amazing!

29

RAW EMOTIONS

These are my original notes I took while going through counseling. These are my real, raw emotions poured out on paper. I only share these because I know others have felt as I did. I want them to know that they are not alone. This is all normal in the process of healing.

November 6, 1990 (original notes)

This was my first day of counseling with Terry. It was kind of scary. I didn't know what to say. She did ask me how I felt about being there. I told her that I didn't know where to start.

I want to take notes so that I can remember what we talked about and what I am finding out about myself. I have asked the Lord to search my heart. He knows me better than I know myself.

He knows why I react the way I do in certain situations, when I don't even know why. There are still a lot of areas in my life that need healing. They are not Christ-like actions. I know that God has gifted people like Terry to help me. So, I have to let go of my huge pride, which is not easy. It means opening up, being honest and being healed. There is always fear of rejection, or being thought of as stupid and maybe laughed at.

Someone, when they heard I was going to counseling, sat me down and told me, "Elaine, you need to forget the past and press forward to what is ahead, leaving the past behind." I kindly told this person that I couldn't leave the past behind and run away from it when it's holding me back from being all God is calling me to be. I explained I was going to face my past and God would bring healing and make me an overcomer. I was done running. I have realized people may say things and think they have your best interest at heart, but what God says to do, you do! The enemy hated what I was doing. After this conversation, I felt a strength I had never had before along with feeling very vulnerable.

Terry asked if I remembered the first time I noticed that something was not right with my mom. I told her the balloon story at the farmhouse. "Elaine, how do you feel when your mom is sick?"

"Nothing was ever explained to us. We thought this was normal behavior, but when I got older and noticed how other families were, I saw that something was not right. I started to be resentful. I became angry at her for the way that she behaved. I was embarrassed. Kids on the school bus would make fun of us. I became angry at God when she was sick. I wondered why God let this happen over and over. He could do something about it, but He didn't. I just figured He didn't care. We were a crazy family. God only cares about normal families. I was so used to people feeling sorry for us. It gave me attention that I didn't have. This was not healthy in me." I asked Terry, ""Why does my mom keep getting sick?"

"Elaine," she said, "We live in a fallen world, full of sin."

I did not like her answer! I asked her again, "But why does this happen over and over?"

Again she answered me, "Elaine, because there is sin in the world." Now I was starting to feel angry, I wanted a REAL fixable answer!

"But, why my mom?" I asked almost in tears.

She looked at me tenderly, "Elaine, there is sin in the world." That time, I heard. I got it. It made sense to me. This simple answer gave me what I was searching for, the why. One more brick was torn down from my wall, but there were many more to go. I shared a lot with Terry; I don't remember everything we talked about. That is why I wanted to journal.

I want to break down this wall I feel around myself. I knew some of the walls were broken down when I let Christ into my heart, but now I needed Him to clean house in my heart. I wanted Him to open up some dirty closets full of hurts that I have tried to pretend didn't happen. Jesus, you need to break down my wall of self-protection and control.

NOVEMBER 20, 1990

Today, Terry and I talked about the rules in my house and family. I explained to her that nobody talked about what was happening and nothing was ever explained to us as kids. We talked in general about Mom's sickness but never about how it was affecting us as kids. I saw what was going on but did not understand why. Maybe I was afraid of what the answer might be if I asked. I wondered if my dad saw how it was affecting us. Did he link our rebellion with what was going on at home? Maybe he didn't know how to talk to us. I wished he would have tried. Because we didn't talk about "it", I wondered if my feelings were real. I felt lonely and unworthy. Maybe I deserved all of this.

I shared with Terry my fear that what happened to Mom could happen to me. I talked about a time when Mom called me when she was sick to tell me she loved me. I was angry because she never told me when she was well, so why now? I thought, Yep, sure you do. I felt very cruel for thinking that way but I wanted her to tell me she loved me when she was well. I realized I was angry because of what I had missed. My relationship with my kids was so different than mine with my mom.

Terry drew things out of me that I had stuffed way down. She made me feel 'normal'. I was finally talking about things I never talked about. And it felt safe.

DECEMBER 4, 1990

Terry asked me to read a book called, "Inside Out". It's about hurt that we bury deep and pretend is not there, although it surfaces in other ways. I think for me it was anger, bitterness, and resentment. I was frustrated at not being able to be in control of certain situations in life. I knew I needed to let God be in control, but I didn't trust Him. This was stopping me from becoming the person in Christ I needed to be.

I don't know if we got anywhere today. I talked about the book. I was having a hard time understanding the right way of thinking. It was different to me. I was seeing there were some things inside of me that were causing fear and problems in my life. I needed to keep going! The book was maybe hitting tender places. I was having a hard time being close with my parents and with my husband for fear of being hurt. I felt I didn't dare to be vulnerable with them, resulting in surface relationships. I wanted deeper relationships. But what if they didn't want that with me? I was afraid of being hurt, afraid of being ignored.

I shared with Terry my frustration of being a wife and a mom. I explained about working part time and that it was easier to be at work where I felt appreciated, but I am overwhelmed with everything there is to do when I come home from work. I told her that I am angry all the time. No one has helped me with all the work at home and taking the kids to all their activities. I confided that at times I feel like I am losing it.

DECEMBER 11.1990
Today, I had a really good day. I had Bible study this morning and a Christmas brunch. We had a good discussion of what the Book of Judges is teaching each of us in our lives.

I then had lunch with my mom and aunt. We talked for two hours. We talked about the Lord the whole time. It was wonderful! I found I had a hard time accepting and respecting what my mom was saying, I think because of past experiences when Mom talked about God. I never knew if what she said was normal or not.

I hope this negative feeling about my mom goes away. I think the more I really get to know my mom, it will, but right now, I need my aunt with me. I watch for my aunt's response to what my mom says to gauge if it's Biblical or not. I feel like I am getting closer to my mom and it is a scary feeling. I feel I am being vulnerable with her. That's good. I want to enjoy spending time with her. I wish I could talk to my mom like I do my aunt.

I feel I got to know my mom a little better today. She told me and her sister something she has never told anyone. It felt good that my mom could do that with me. My mom struggled with her own relationship with her mother. My aunt, my mom's sister, shared today that Grandma didn't believe in telling her children that she loved them or that they looked nice or that they were doing a good job. She thought that you might make your children vain.

My mom thought her parents didn't set a good Christian example. Yes, they were believers, but maybe never understood the personal relationship with Christ. They were legalistic and didn't understand the personal relationship with Christ. They did not teach their children this, but we were not taught that either. My mom and my aunt felt their parents didn't know the love of Christ, so they could not give it to their children. Denominations were important to them and you married someone in your own denomination. I remember my grandmother asking me where Kenny went to church; I told her it was the same one I went to. "Oh good!" she said.

I think my mom had some of the same feelings her parents had. This conversation helped me to understand my mom a lot and some of the things she said to us. I didn't blame her or my grandparents. I loved my grandmother and always felt loved by her. I think she had softened through the years. My mom has changed a lot in the last couple of years. I have watched her grow in the Lord. She became born again later in life. She told her sister about it. If my mom would have told me about being born again while I was still living at home, I would have thought it was another one of her crazy ideas only because I didn't know about it.

I so want to be healed from how I feel when my mom is sick. I hate this in myself. Some of those old feelings for my mom are still there. I want them gone! I know I need to go through a healing process and this is all a part of it. I want and need to get rid of the garbage. I need to learn to accept people where they are in life. God is in control of their lives, not me. I just need to be there to love them, to put my arms around them when they are going through rough times, even if I don't understand. I NEED to accept the fact that mental illness is a fact of life, just like cancer and other illnesses. It's nothing to be ashamed of.

DECEMBER 19, 1990

I am writing this on Thursday and I had counseling on Tuesday. She asked me how my week went and I told her it had its ups and downs. On the way to counseling that morning, I was listening to a tape on mental illness and manic depression. She asked me how I felt when I was listening to it. There was part of me that wanted to shut it off. It was painful to hear. Each thing that was said on the tape, I had seen my mom go through.

One thing I am learning about myself is that I demand a better life. Sometimes I think my ways are better than God's. Look what He did with my mom. For some reason, I think I deserve a life without any pain or misery. I had enough of that growing up. God should make my life better, but He probably won't. I am finding that I really am a demanding person. When things don't go the way that I think they should, I am very angry at the person, even God, for messing things up for the so-called perfect life that I want. This demanding spirit in me is a great sin and causes a lot of problems in my life. I need to repent so that I can grow more in my walk with the Lord or my spiritual growth will be stunted.

For the next two weeks, Terry wants me to really look at why I get angry at my husband and the kids. What is my motive behind what I say to them? I know I have selfish motives. I want them to fit into this perfect life I want. I am learning that I need to let God take charge of every area of my life. I need to let go and trust God. His plans and ways are different than mine.

This is something I got out of the book, "Inside Out" by Larry Crabb:

"I know my ways seem to ignore your concerns at times. I want you to trust Me when you feel unusually tired and I call on you to get up. I want you to trust Me when you're eager to serve and I put you on hold. But you will never learn to trust Me until you come to terms with my authority. Trust will never emerge from a demanding spirit. Let's start with a clear understanding: I give the orders. You do what you are told. With that as a beginning, you will eventually taste my goodness and the rich fellowship with Me and come to trust Me deeply."

This really showed me how tight of a hold I still wanted on my own life and that I really was not trusting in God. Nor do I trust God with the people in my life. What made me think I could do a better job than God? I was making a mess! I am so glad God knows me better than I know me. I am so glad He is showing me where I need to change. I am so thankful He opened my eyes and heart to want to change. "Lord, always let my heart and mind be open to hearing Your voice. Help me to be obedient to what You want me to do. Not my will Lord, but Yours."

JANUARY 15, 1991

We had snow last week so I missed counseling. It's been a while. I have been reading a book called, "Co-Dependent No More". Boy, did I see myself! A co-dependent person is one who has let another person's behavior affect him or her, and who is obsessed with controlling that person's behavior. The co-dependent does more than their share of work then resents those they feel should be doing this work. They feel angry, victimized, unappreciated, and used.

Terry asked me how I did this in my family. I told her when my girls fight over clothes, there is a war. I hate it and get frustrated. Terry suggested I sit down with the girls and have them decide what they will let each other wear and come up with some kind of agreement. If one breaks the agreement, there will be consequences. I will make a rule that each girl is not allowed to go into the other's room without permission.

I talked with her about my frustration and anger with the lack of help and support. When I come home from work, everyone just sits back and expects me to do everything. And I let them! Then I get angry. I don't know if I get angrier at myself or my family. I trained them. I feel like a martyr when I say, "Fine, I will do it." I then wait for them to feel sorry for me. It never happens.

One day, Ken and the kids had been home an hour before me and were watching TV when I walked in the door from work. "Where is dinner? What is for dinner?" they all asked me.

"You didn't start it?" I asked them.

"You're supposed to make it." they all replied back to me. I went into the kitchen and started to make dinner. No, I thought. Nothing is going to change around here unless I change first. I had talked to my family about helping out more and that I was going to be putting in a long day at work, something I rarely did. They all looked at me like I was from another planet. I made a light dinner for myself then headed to bed.

"What about our dinner?"

"Your dad will make you dinner or you can. You are old enough," I called back to them. I lay on the bed exhausted from the day and listened

to my family trying to figure out what they were going to do; they were not happy. They ended up going out to eat.

I wasn't sure I had done the right thing, but Terry told me I had. I am learning to step out of my co-dependent role and it's rocking the boat at home. I am handing them responsibilities they are very capable of doing. It was just easier for me to do it myself before. This is hard work, holding to what I say. They don't like the change, but that is not my problem. I am going to need a lot of strength from God to stay this course. I want to teach my kids responsibility for their own actions and not blame other people or expect others to do things for them even if it's hard. Hard is not bad. I have to learn to give them back their responsibilities in love, not anger. I need to step back from situations instead of thinking I am the rescuer trying to fix everything. This is not easy for me to do. But I am starting. If I don't change, neither will anyone else. I hope the damage I have done is not beyond repair. "Lord, heal my kids where I mess up."

After six months of counseling one-on-one with Terry, she encouraged me to join a group counseling she was leading. I went for a few months and listened to others share their lives and struggles. I personally didn't feel it was helpful after a few times of attending. I wanted to move on and felt like the group was stuck in talking about all the hard things in their lives. I wanted to know how to overcome them. When one person was sharing about her dog's death, I had had enough. Maybe it was God's way of moving me on.

I was thankful for what Terry had taught me and the insight I gained through my time with her. Different people are a part of our growing process. I did not want to be one of the people who was in counseling for two years or more. I wanted to move forward, not stay stagnant talking about my problems all the time. I wanted to be like a river, always moving forward, not like a pond, staying in one place with scum collected around the edge. I wanted to get over 'me'! More of You, Lord Jesus, and less of me! This was the desire of my heart. I am not there yet.

30
PLEASE GOD, NOT AGAIN!

These are more notes from my journal.

February 25, 1992

A friend of mine, who works at the rest home where my mom volunteers, told me that my mom quit. One of my siblings explained that mom seemed depressed. My mind started to panic and I felt sick inside. I didn't want to think about it. Maybe my mom's medication just went haywire or something. I will see my mom tomorrow. Do I ask my her how she is doing? Do I bring up quitting the rest home? No! I am afraid. I will see if Mom brings it up. I don't want this illness to happen to my mom again! I hate all the feelings that come up from this place in me where I stash them. I start to feel hate. I can't seem to separate Mom from her illness. I need to hate the sickness, not my mom. What is wrong with me? I am feeling anxious inside and weak. Maybe I should go back to the counselor. "Lord, the way you teach us hope and life are through trials. I want to learn!"

February 26, 1992

Mom was really quiet today at lunch. "Mom, is there anything new you would like to tell us?" I asked her.

"No," she replied back. Why didn't she tell me? She never talks to me! What is going on inside of her? Does Dad notice anything? My grandma, my aunt, as well as a friend of my mom's noticed my mom was not herself.

Mom didn't smile or laugh today. This sets off alarms in me. My grandmother shared with me that she is worried about Mom. "This hurts to see her like this," my grandma said to me. I let her know it affects us all, but that maybe Mom was just having a bad day. "No, I don't think so," Grandma said worriedly.

I called my dad this evening and asked him how he thought Mom was doing. "It will be ok, Elaine, I will take care of things," he told me.

"Dad, I am not a little girl anymore. Please don't hide things from me. I want you to tell me the truth about how Mom is doing."

"She is fine," my dad assured me, yet I heard the pain in his voice. He hung up hurriedly so that I wouldn't have a chance to say more.

My aunt shared with me today her worry also about my mom. She doesn't want this to happen again either. "I have felt close to her the last couple of years. We were starting to have fun together as sisters," my aunt told me. This is the first time I have heard others voice to me how my mom's illness affects them. On the bottom of my journal book on this page is, **"Trust in the Lord with all your heart, and lean not on your own understanding. In all your ways acknowledge Him, and He will make straight your paths." (Proverbs 3:5, 6, ESV)**

March 28, 1992

Mom is still not doing well. I don't feel like talking to Kenny about Mom. He might not understand why I feel inside the way I do right now. What if he doesn't really listen? Then I will feel really stupid that I shared my feelings. I don't want my mom's sickness to ruin my family life. I want to keep it as far away as I can from my home. I hurt for my dad. I wish I could hurt for my mom. What is wrong with me? I only feel anger. When will this anger go away? There is so much pain attached to this illness! "Help me, God!"

I called my friend, Ann, who works at the mental health clinic. She shared with me what she legally could. "Elaine, your mom knows she is going through a depression. She made an appointment to come back. We did increase her medication." What my friend told me, reassured me. I just wish I had a better attitude toward my mom. There is still a little girl in me who is afraid of being hurt. I feel walls of protection all around me. "Lord, You need to help me tear down these walls! I know You are with me and will help me." Today, the bottom of my journal page read: **"Oh, give thanks to the LORD! Call upon His name!" (Psalm 105:1, ESV)**

Those are the only entries I put in my journal when my mom was ill again. Sometimes it's too painful to write.

Elaine Oostra

31
GOD REVEALS MY HEART

My journaling continued.

February 6, 1995

Even though I am no longer in counseling, I find journaling helps. The first step to healing is acknowledging there is a problem. It's been two years since the last episode of my mom's illness. I wonder if I will handle it differently, if it happens again, than I have in the past. I thought once I was saved, I would handle it better. I haven't, but now that I have gone through counseling, maybe I will. The nightmares I had of my mom's illness before I was saved have stopped.

One of my siblings called me as I was writing this. "Mom seemed different when I talked to her on the phone this morning. She said she wasn't doing really well." I confirmed that I did notice Mom was overly sensitive today at lunch. This is not good, I thought to myself. Maybe Mom is just sad over losing her mom recently. Maybe that is all it is. "Lord, let this be all that it is, please!" But I knew. I saw the warning signs too many times when the illness would make its entrance into our lives. *"Help me be sensitive to my mother's hurts. Oh Lord, the pain is so great within me! There still is a need in me to have my mom well. I need to feel this pain that I keep shoving down inside of me. Why is this pain still here? I am angry at what this illness does to our family."* I cried from deep within my soul. The tears came.

February 19, 1995

At the age of thirty-eight, I really understand that there is pain in my life. I still get angry in my mom's presence. How can I separate her from her illness? It's so hard for me to do this.

"Why God? I want my mom to stop this from progressing. Why can't she? What goes on inside her head? Why can't I have more compassion for her? God, I hate how I feel! Please heal me, change me! I have to look at what my mom is going through. This is hard for me, but I have to. She feels, she hurts. God, You will be with us through all this pain that will come again."

I can't take personally what my mom says to me right now. I just had a phone conversation with her. I hung up the phone and cried. She wouldn't say these things to me if she was well. Why does she treat me this way when she is sick? It's hard sometimes to remember it's the mental illness that is speaking, not her. ""God, this is hard! Help me with this, God." I know I have to 'feel' in order to bring healing. What is inside of me has to come to the surface. I have to give God all the pain that is within me. How else can I get rid of it? "I keep giving it to You God , will it ever go away? I thought being a Christian would help me to be able to handle this the way a "good Christian" should. It doesn't make it any easier. There are no answers. God, You promised to give me strength each day. I can't look past today. It's too wearing. It hurts, God. It hurts so badly!"

I have a hard time being with my mom, even looking at her. I just want to ignore her right now. Memories come pouring into my brain. I can't stop them. They make me sad. All the signs that come each time my mom gets sick are showing their ugly heads once again. Each time, I pray it's the last time. Right now, I am deflated. I know what is to come once again. "Lord, give me strength to be around my mom. I can't do this on my own. I am weak. You promise to make me strong when I feel faint. I confess the feeling of hate toward my mom, of anger toward her. Help me, Lord. I feel so powerless!"

Does she feel powerless? Why don't I even want to look at how she feels? What are my fears? I am seeing my mom today. "I need You to forgive me, Lord, for this destructive anger in me, for the way I treat my mom and my attitude toward her." This is what I didn't even want to face. I need to confront me! As long as I can blame Mom, I don't have to look at the bitterness that has been growing for years in me and the effect it has had on me as a mom and wife. My mom didn't ask for this illness, so why am I so angry at her?

"God, I look at my anger and it's at You for allowing this horrible illness in my mom that affects us all. How do I forgive You? You are God! You could have stopped it! I have blamed You for so long, I see I still do. How can I feel forgiveness for You when I am angry at you? Help me to understand why You allowed this. Are You teaching me to trust You and to learn unconditional love? I see I don't trust You, God. Lord, keep teaching me to trust You. Help me to grow. What do You want me to learn? Teach me to love You. I read in Your word that we will have trials in life. Everything that comes into my life is first filtered through Your fingers of love. My head knows this, but my heart needs to receive this! Lord God, I am afraid to relinquish my whole heart to You. There are still walls of self-protection around my heart. Heal me, oh God! This is the cry of my heart! I can't heal my own heart. I can hide nothing from You, nothing! Everything on the outside can look perfect to others, but inside, it's rotten. I am so tired of pretense. Am I supposed to smile through all of this? Where are you? Aren't You supposed to be a God more powerful than all Satan's destruction that he pours out upon me?"

I Corinthians 10:13 says, "God is faithful, and will not let you be tempted beyond your ability, but with the temptation he will also provide you the way of escape, that you may be able to endure it."(ESV)

"Does this apply only to the times when I am tempted by sinful desires? Is that the only time that You will provide a way out or that You will help me to bear in the time of temptations? Lord, when I go through trials, I am tempted, tempted to give up on You, tempted to curse You for what I am going through, when I don't understand, and I

am angry that You won't change what is hurting me so badly. Does this qualify as a sinful situation? Does this qualify as a being tempted beyond what I can bear? The word "bear" means strength. You have promised me strength to give me joy in my trials, for who I am in you. I don't have to be joyful about all of the yucky stuff going on around me. That is such a relief! David in the Psalms felt forgotten by You at times, yet he trusted You and Your unfailing love. So, I will trust in Your unfailing love. You put Your righteousness to the test. You are not always going to change my circumstances that are trying to devour me, but You will never leave me nor forsake me. This is where my hope comes from. I don't belong in this world. I am an alien here. I belong to You, God."

"Oh, my sweet daughter, Elaine. You are learning to cry out to Me. You are learning to trust Me with your heart and this pleases Me. You are right, I see it all and yet I love you unconditionally. I will not pressure you to give Me your whole heart. I will wait patiently as I reveal to you each corner hidden in your heart that I will heal. Time is nothing to Me. Just keep crying out to Me to heal the bitterness inside of you. Be perseverant. This will mature you and complete you so you will lack in nothing. My joy will be found complete in you. Patience, dear child."

Note: As I read back on my journal, I understand now that what I felt was normal. I have many Christian female friends in their 70's watching their husbands' health and memory fail. I listen as they talk about their frustration at their husbands, then feeling so guilty about the anger or shortness they express at their spouses. They are angry at what is happening and they can't stop it. All the while, deep down, their frustration is at the health issue, not their husbands. But they, like I did, are having a hard time separating the person from the failing body. It's so hard to watch someone who used to be strong become physically weak. I see adult children caring for an aging parent whose memory is failing and losing patience with them, and then feeling guilty. I felt so abnormal for years in the feelings I had toward my mom and Satan loved to condemn me, even using other people's mouths to fulfill his purpose. I am not justifying how I felt. It's a part of human nature. I have just learned to take those feelings to God and ask Him to heal me where I needed to be healed. I am who God says I am, not who others 'think' I am.

Elaine Oostra

32
BITTERROOTS

The word 'bitterroot' seemed to resonate inside of me. I came across it many times as I studied the Bible. I had avoided it long enough; it was time to deal with it.

It's really hard to look in a mirror and see the truth about yourself. How long have I walked around with broccoli stuck between my teeth? I can feel it, but think, 'I will deal with it later', only to forget about it until someone says, "Um, you might want to brush or get a toothpick." I had bitterness seeping out of me, but I was pretending it wasn't there, like broccoli stuck between my teeth. God, with His Word, was showing me my bitterness. I had been crying out to God to change me. I was tired of being bitter, I wanted to be better. Besides, my bitter fruit was getting rancid and pretty rotten!

Ephesians 4:31-5:2 describes a bitterroot the best to me. "Let all bitterness and wrath and anger and clamor and slander be put away from you along with malice. Be kind to one another, tenderhearted, forgiving one another, as Christ in God forgave you. Therefore be imitators of God, as beloved children. And walk in love, as Christ loved us and gave himself up for us, a fragrant offering and sacrifice to God." (ESV)

Have you ever seen a person who is mad all the time and if they might smile, their face would surely crack? You can see the anger in their eyes, and in the lines of the face, even if the person is young. You can hear it in the tone of a voice. You can hear it when they protest that they are not bitter. There is even enjoyment in holding things against others. A bitterroot bears fruit. It is bitter fruit. This described me!

The temptation in my life was to always look at what the offender, my mom's illness, had done to me. I used to think I wasn't bitter, I was just easily hurt. Even if my mom never got sick again, I was still angry about the illness and how it affected me.

Bitterness was not based upon what the other person did at all. It was the result of what I did and who I was. My mom's illness just revealed what was inside of my heart. The only way to get rid of this bitterness was to call it what it was, 'sin.' "God forgive me. My head knows this. God, help my heart to receive this. Change me, God!"

How do I forgive my mom when she didn't ask for this illness? How do I forgive the illness? If bitterness comes from unforgiveness which then causes anger issues, I am not bringing about the life that God desires. "Lord God, take away my pride that stops me from really seeing my sin. This is hard! I don't like what I see in me! But I hate this pride in me, I hate it!"

"Search me, O God, and know my heart! Try me and know my thoughts! See if there be any grievous way in me, and lead me in the way everlasting!" (Psalm 139:23-24, ESV)

This is the cry of my heart. I wanted the memories of my past to change me for the better. I was so tired of being bitter and angry. I wanted to get better. I was full of fear and I lacked trust.

My walls that I thought would protect me from getting hurt were killing me, emotionally and spiritually. I read and studied the Word diligently, but I saw I was not letting it change me. *"O God, I want it to. God I want to trust You and I don't."*

I saw I was so insecure. I wanted to fill up this emptiness in me. I thought my husband would fill it, but if there was an emptiness in him and he was looking for me to fill his emptiness, then we were two empty, insecure, married people looking for each other to fulfill each other's needs. What a pair we were!

I thought having kids would fill this need in me. The demands of raising kids were great and it made it harder for me to cope. I thought having a new house, furniture, and a job would fill me.

Remember, I am a saved, messed up person. God took me as I was. He was cleaning me up. Before I was saved, I did not see my sin of bitterness, but I sure did now. I had needs that needed to be met. I was insecure and frazzled. I was a selfish person.

"Lord, I confess and repent of this. I confess my attitudes. I can dress nice, put on my makeup and look good to everyone. The need to 'appear' together and happy in front of others is nothing but stinking pride in me. You, O God, know what is in my heart. How do you still love me? Thank You for Your unconditional love for me. Please help me to love as You love!"

Elaine Oostra

33
THE MOVE TO IDAHO IN 1998

Two of our daughters were now married and Ken and I had one grandchild. God was in the process of preparing me for a change in life and in my heart.

Something in that previous year had felt unsettled and unsatisfying. For the last 12 years, I worked in two different gift shops as a manager. I was starting to feel trapped. I had been doing Precept Bible Study for over 15 years and asking God, *"How can I share with others all that I have learned from Your Word, God?"* I didn't want to stop studying; I just wanted to pour out what God poured into me. I did lead a Precepts study as well as a few light Bible studies. I led a young girls' group at church and did volunteer counseling at an unwed mothers' home. However, I found myself asking God, *"What do You want to do with my life? Is this it?"*

Our youngest daughter was a sophomore in high school. She had switched high schools at the beginning of the year. We moved from the farm that we sold, into one of the spec houses Ken had built, which was in a different school district.

I think Ken was feeling like me, anticipating a change, except he wanted to move to a drier climate. I did not want to move! I just wanted 'something' different. Ken was building spec houses as well as custom farming, putting up feed for local farmers. One of our main farming customers moved to Idaho. This got Ken to check out farming there.

When I asked God to heal my heart, I had no idea how He was going to do it. I thought he would just 'heal it'. God knew each day of my life before I was even born. He knew each detail. He knew when and how He would bring healing into my life. I didn't and it's a good thing, I may have objected to His plan. God needed to *uproot* me in more ways than one.

Ken left in March for Idaho to check out crop farming. "When are you coming home?" I asked him. He had been gone for a month.

"It's been raining here and we can't get into the fields," he told me. A month later, we had the same conversation. In the middle of May, he came home for the weekend, for our son's wedding.

Our 25th anniversary was coming up on June 8th. Ken wanted me to drive the 580 miles to Idaho so we could be together. I did. I had flown up once to see where he was. I thought Southern Idaho was the ugliest place on earth. It was all desert and the mountains were bald! What they called trees, I called shrubs. How can there be any Christians here? "If you think I am moving here, you're wrong!" I told Ken.

Each time Ken and I talked, he would mention maybe moving there. Something in me was unsettled about the future. I think I was fearful. *"Lord, I am hip deep in solid cement firm around me in Washington. I don't want to leave my kids, my new granddaughter, all of our family. Lord Jesus, if You want us to move then You will have to break up the concrete around me, because I don't want to move!"* I prayed this, kneeling by my couch. I thought there would be no way our youngest daughter would want to switch again to another high school. I decided if she wouldn't move, I wouldn't move. I would just stay in Washington until she graduated. Ken would just have to go back and forth if he wanted to move to Idaho. I had settled it in my mind. I thought it was safe to throw out a fleece to God, *"If our daughter wants to move, I will move. If she doesn't want to move, I know we are not supposed to."* I told no one of my fleece.

The next morning I drove my daughter to the high school. For some reason, she was sitting in the back seat, maybe to get a little more sleep. "Honey, I need to talk to you about something. Dad is not sure when he is coming home from Idaho and he really likes it there. Now I am going to say something to you, and you can honestly tell me how you feel." I was sure she would be mad. "Dad is seriously thinking about moving to Idaho, but we don't have to….." I didn't even get to finish what I wanted to say.

My daughter popped up from the back seat, "Really? Are you serious?" I looked in the rearview mirror, expecting to see an angry face. Instead, I saw a smile from one side of her face to the other! "I want to move! When are we going?" she excitedly asked me.

"Wait a minute. This means you have to go to another school, again. You really don't want to do this!"

"Yes, I do Mom, I don't like this school. I want to move to Idaho!"

The cement, my comfort zone that I had firmly planted myself in, was cracking around me into little pieces. At 43 years old, the thought of starting all over in a strange land scared me and excited me at the same time. I felt like Abram in the Bible.

"Now the LORD had said to Abram, 'Go from your country (in my case, state), your kindred and your father's house, (*my family*) to the land that I will show you.'" Verse 4a states "So Abram went, as the LORD had told him". (Genesis 12:1, 4a ESV)

He gathered all of his things and left! I am not like Abram, but maybe his wife was like me. They did get to take people with them. I was just taking my youngest and my husband and leaving two married daughters, a granddaughter, and a son and new daughter-in-law. I was also leaving a grandparent, parents, siblings, cousins and life-time friends. I was a family-oriented person who was now going to where I knew no one!

Then, I saw in verse 1 of Genesis 12 that God told Abram, "I will show you." The unsettled feeling in me was settled. We would be moving. *"Lord Jesus, I am asking you to go before me to this new place. I don't know anyone. I ask you to put **friends** in my life and to find us **a home**. I don't want to hop from church to **church**. Show us where you want us to go. Everything in Idaho is so brown. Can you find me a house with trees and green and possibly a water view of some kind?"* Abram was a little more trusting than I was.

If you know the full story of Abram to Abraham in Genesis, you know God did more than just move him geographically. God had a plan.

I love the examples God gives us in His Word to encourage us. It still pertains to us today. God was taking me from the green, lush mountains, lakes, and ocean, into the desert to heal my heart. He heard my cry. I am so excited to tell you, but I have other stories I need to tell you first. It's like a puzzle. All of the pieces have to be patiently put together to see the whole picture. Each piece of the puzzle has part of the story. If you leave one piece out of the picture, the story is incomplete.

Well, God moved me, more than geographically. God had a plan!

34
MY FRIEND, ANN

I believe God places people in our lives sometimes to help us grow, to see the gift of life through other people's eyes when our view has become so distorted.

Ann and I got to know each other in our later 30's. Our husbands were friends and fished together. We then started to go out to dinner as couples. Ann and I hit it off. We started to do things together with our families, like camping and going to the ocean. The guys would fish and we would play. Ann worked as a mental health nurse at the same clinic where my mom was treated. She knew my mom and at times would reassure me of my mom's care. It was a comfort to me knowing Ann was there.

Ann, to me, was a picture of calm in a storm. Nothing seemed to ruffle her. She always had a peace about her. She never yelled at her kids like I did. She always spoke calmly. I wanted that character quality. Her sense of humor was what I enjoyed the most because I didn't really have this. I was way too serious and uptight compared to her.

Ann took up running and wanted me to join her. I was 39 and never ran before. On one of our ocean camping trips, Ann challenged me to run the beach with her. I made it a mile each day we were there. When we got home, she wanted to start running every day with me, but I told her I needed to work up to the three miles she was doing so I could keep up and I would let her know when I was ready.

For a week, I ran by myself until I could do three miles. I was proud of myself! I was learning to conquer things in my life that I thought I couldn't do.

We met often in a wooded park near us at 6 a.m. Trails were through the whole woods as many used this for running. I grew to love running. The air was clean and seemed to fill me with energy.

When the weather was bad, we would run in town. Ann loved to be silly. On one of our runs, we headed over to the rest home. I followed her most of the time. She ran off the sidewalk, onto the yard surrounding the rest home, past all the windows of the residents there, waving at them. She wanted to run down the hallway and I said, "No!" She loved to run through the alleys and make all the sensor lights go off and get the dogs barking while it was still dark out. She had a humorous mischievousness about her in many ways. There are many stories I could tell on her.

One time we ran a five-mile fun run in town. We both had the same time in the run. Ann won the 40-year-old bracket. I was going to be 40 in a few weeks so I didn't get a medal around my neck. I kidded her that I was going to steal it. I earned it just as much as she did! We joked about it. Other runners told us we ran in perfect step together. We had been running daily so it was natural.

Ann taught me how to laugh, especially at myself. She taught me to see the humor in so many areas I took way too seriously. She brought joy into my life. She helped me to be a better mom and wife. I had a long ways to go in improving in these areas of my life.

One morning, I vented to Ann as we began our run through the woods. I told her that my mom was sick again and I was mad. Through tears and anger, I told Ann everything I was mad about concerning my mom and my hatred for her illness. At this time, I could not separate the illness from my mom.

"Well, at least your mom is alive!" she yelled at me. I stopped in my tracks, I had never heard Ann yell.

I yelled back, "What good is it? Look at what she does! I want her to be well. I want God to heal her!"

"You have a mom!" she yelled back at me. "Mine is gone and I miss her. Appreciate your mom while you still have her," she told me through her tears. Ann's parents were killed in a head-on collision when she was just 30 years old.

I wish I could say that day changed my heart and I saw the light. It didn't. I did see the pain my friend had in her own life. I apologized to her. It brought us closer. Ann and I started praying for our kids and husbands on our runs. We prayed for our health and thanked God for healthy bodies.

We took a road trip to California with no kids, a couples getaway. On this trip, I noticed something about Ann's speech; she seemed to slur. We even kidded about it. I thought no more about it. We were having a wonderful time driving to the coast.

When Ann returned to work, one of her co-workers asked if she had had a stroke. They noticed a change in her speech. This alarmed her and she went to a doctor who performed many tests.

Ken and I got a call from Ben saying they wanted to come over and talk to us. It was discovered that Ann had Lou Gehrig's disease, also known as ALS. None of us really understood what this would bring. It was life-changing news no one wanted to hear. There was no cure. This disease slowly weakens the muscles in the body. Ann had upper body ALS, and was given two years to live. Slowly it became harder and harder for her to speak.

It was in-between this time that Ken and I moved to Idaho. It was one of the most difficult decisions we have ever made. We talked in depth with Ben and Ann about our move. We would stay, if they wanted us to. We had promised Ann we would never desert her through this illness. She reminded me of this when we told her of our plans. God's plans are, at times, really different than ours.

I am learning not to make promises. We only hurt people. We don't know the future, only He does. Things change. We told her we would come to visit as often as we could, and we did. Ann even drove to Idaho with her daughter. She knew of a faith healer near where we lived. It turned out to be a person just wanting to take advantage of people like her for money. That is another story in itself that I won't get into. At least I got to spend time with her.

On one of my visits to see Ann, we spent a day at a friend's house overlooking the bay. I have a picture of us sitting in rockers by the big bay window looking at the water. The ALS had greatly affected her ability to talk. Eating became more difficult. Weight was dropping off her body. Our days of running were only a memory. When I came up, we walked through the wooded paths, me silently crying behind her holding onto her portable oxygen tank. Her speech was pretty much gone.

When Ken was able to go up to Washington after haying, we would spend hours playing card games with Ann and Ben. Ann could still laugh and be her mischievous self. She would have us all in stitches, laughing as she hid the main cards.

We planned another trip together as couples. Tickets were bought for Hawaii. I bought insurance for the first time, in case we needed to cancel. A week or two before the trip, Ben rushed Ann to the emergency room. She could no longer breathe on her own. The effects of the disease had become more apparent and life threatening. We canceled the trip we were all looking so forward to. Ken and I went to Washington to visit them instead of Hawaii.

I had not seen Ann for about a month and a half or more. I was shocked when I saw her. She had a tracheotomy as well as a feeding tube. The reality of my dying friend hit me. I was losing her. Ann had a machine she could type on and it would speak out her words through her machine.

She would "talk" of being healed. I told her I knew God could heal her too, but God did not give me the reassurance that it would be on this earth. I would not speak something to her that God did not tell me to say. If God healed her on this earth, that would be awesome! If God took her to be with Him, this disease would not be going with her. She would be totally healed. God knew before she was born her number of days on this earth.

There were times we could talk about her death and funeral. We would laugh about what I would dress her in. She had these funky, flashy, running pants that I threatened to put on her. She thought it would be great for everyone to see her dressed like that.

We knew our time was getting shorter with her. I think we all cried an ocean full since we heard the dreaded news. I was working at a bank when I informed my boss that my friend was dying and when that day happened, I was going to Washington. She could fire me if she liked. I just wanted her to know ahead of time. It was not easy getting off work. I had a hard enough time using sick days when I was sick. I just went to work; I didn't want to leave everyone shorthanded. But this was different.

Ken and I were planning another trip up to Washington when Ben called telling us she was getting worse. I assured him we were going to be there in a few days. I had already arranged for the time off work. *Oh, God, please wait, I want to see her one more time!*

I came home for my lunch break thinking, *One more day and we are leaving for Washington, I can't wait!* The phone rang, I got it because Ken was busy talking to the insurance man that was at our house.

"Ann is gone," I heard Ben say.

"What? What do you mean she's gone?" Panic set in my body.

The soft weak voice again told me Ann was gone. "It's over."

"No!" I screamed into the phone. "No! I am coming! She can't be gone, I am coming! You're wrong!" I yelled at him. I fell to the floor, crying, with the receiver in my lap. "No, no, no!"

It felt like every muscle in my body left me. Ken took the phone. The insurance man left. I heard Ken tell Ben we were on our way. I was numb with shock. We both were. Ken and I packed our things and left. I made him call my boss to tell her the news.

After the funeral, Ben had the hearse go through the park that Ann and I ran through for six years. He did this for me. He had asked for permission. There had been a bad wind storm and a lot of branches had fallen, but the park keeper let us go through, maybe out of guilt for yelling at us. Ann and I had always somehow seemed to get in trouble with this park keeper. Ann would sneak her dog in with no leash and we always got caught.

As some of us followed in cars behind the hearse, we noticed branches stuck underneath and they were being dragged through the whole park. They dropped out once we left the park. We all laughed and said, "Ann, you did it again!" I know it's silly, but it was like it was her goodbye to us and she was still her silly self in heaven. It's funny how sad you can be and yet have laughter.

Ben asked me if there was anything of Ann's that I wanted. I said, "Yes." I went into their bedroom and hanging on the mirror was the plastic gold medal we, I thought, both had won. I smiled with tears and put it around my neck. It was full of memories.

I know she will greet me when I enter into heaven. She went to be with Jesus when she was only 46. I am long past that age. I will never forget what she taught me through her life: the gift of laughter.

35
HOME, CHURCH, FRIENDS

HOME

We bought an older home in Parma, Idaho with two huge sycamore trees in the front and one huge walnut tree in the back. Across the street was a lush green city park with a small irrigation ditch that flows through it and a city pool. God has a sense of humor. I had prayed for a water view and trees.

Even though we were looking for farmland, we ended up in town. Every farm property we looked at sold before we could even put an offer on it. We later bought 60 acres which we rented. We have lived in the same house since we moved to Idaho. We have done a lot of renovating. I love decorating. God had a purpose for the home we bought.

Before we moved to Idaho, I had prayed and asked God to show me who He created me to be. I felt like I was always trying to live up to others' expectations of who they thought I was, or maybe who I thought I should be. It was tiring.

God has given me a ministry of ministering to teen girls and I love it! During the school year, for over fourteen years now, on Tuesday mornings from 7 a.m. to almost 8 a.m., high school girls come over for a Bible study in my front room. I serve them juice and cinnamon rolls and sticky buns with great delight. I also started a girls Bible study group on Monday evenings that includes dinner. The girls get cozy by the fireplace and on my couches and we study God's Word together. I also have hosted other women's Bible studies in this home.

Before I moved to Idaho, I was always afraid to have people in my home. I thought I couldn't be a good hostess. I was so intimidated by women who could cook lovely meals and have a beautifully set table. I have learned a Biblical hostess is different than someone who is an entertaining hostess. You just have to love on people and have an open home. It's that simple.

I wonder how many women like me don't feel their home is good enough or don't have matching dishes and this stops them from inviting people into their homes. I loved going to a friend's house where crumbs on the floor crunched under my feet as we made our way to her couch. I didn't come to judge her home; I came because of the love that flowed from her.

CHURCH

I didn't want to church hop. The first Sunday my daughter and I were in Parma, we wondered where we would go to church. Ken wasn't able to go with us because of field work so it was left up to us. There was a church a block from our house, but we noticed no cars and it was getting late. We found out later that they were having their church picnic in the park.

I said to my daughter, "I saw a Baptist church down the country road where your dad was working. Let's go find it. At least we know what Baptists believe."

As we pulled into the parking lot of what I thought was the Baptist church, I saw the sign and said, "This is a Presbyterian Church. Oh well, let's try it." Silently I prayed and asked God to show me if this was where we were supposed to be and if not, to make it very clear to me. I did not know anything about

Presbyterians. We were a little late. As we walked down the aisle to find a seat, we were greeted by the pastor in front of everyone in this small country church. The rest of the congregation got up and shook hands with those around them. In front of me was a lady and as I held her hand, she touched my heart. *"Lord, I want to get to know this lady!"*

"You will," I heard Him say to me.

"But how?" I asked Him.

"Don't worry, you will." The sermon that Sunday felt like it was just for me and it answered many questions I had about this church. I didn't 'accidentally' pull into the wrong parking lot. **God had a plan** in the church we still attend to this day.

After we lived in Parma for two years, I became the youth leader at church. I love teaching teens. God used this time to bring healing into my life. Two incidents, one little and one huge and life changing, happened while teaching the teens.

In one of the nine years I was a youth leader, I taught the Ten Commandments. When we came to "Thou shall not steal," I was deeply convicted, especially after the girl that was helping me told the teens a story of when she had stolen something and then years later paid back the money. Since I had been saved, I had thought many times about that maternity top I had stolen when I was going to marry Ken and the barrettes I had stolen for my wedding. The guilt had been weighing heavily on me for many years, yet I was too embarrassed to say to the store owner, "Hey by the way, when I was a stupid teen, I stole from you!" I thought of sending cash without putting my name on the envelope. I worried what the store owner would think of me; I knew their whole family.

Guilt is good. I had a conscience. It meant I knew I was guilty and I needed to take care of it. In front of the whole youth group I said, "Hey guys, I have a confession to make…" I told them the whole story. "I want you all to hold me accountable. I am going to write a letter to the store owners and send them a check. Next week when we come back together, I want you to ask me if I did it." They did and I was able to tell them that I had written the check.

A few weeks later, I got a letter back. They no longer had the store. They thanked me for the money and the confession. I had written about the teens that I was teaching and how God had convicted me. They used the money to buy Bibles for people who didn't have one. I read this letter to the youth group. I talked to them about sin catching up to you and how it stays with you unless you take care of it. The guilt that I could have gotten rid of years ago was finally gone. The memory that plagued me for years was now replaced with God's forgiving grace.

FRIENDS

As faithful as God was in giving us a home and a church, He was also putting amazing women in my life. The lady I met at church and wanted to know, I met again at a Bible study later that week. A woman my age came up to me the first Sunday in Idaho and invited me to a Bible study at her house. I was so excited to meet new women. When I got there, I saw her. Her name was Barb. She came up to me and asked me about myself. For some reason, I told her I had done many Precept Bible Studies. She grabbed me and said, "I know why you are here!"

"You do?" I asked, puzzled.

"Yes! I have been praying for someone who knows about Precepts!" she said. "God brought you here!" Barb became my first faithful friend. She is still so dear to me today. She would call me a couple of times a week my first year in Parma. She would ask how I was doing and I would just start crying. I was so homesick. I missed my grandchild; it was like being away from my own baby. I missed my daughters, our family, and my close friends. I missed going into a store and knowing people and them knowing me. I missed the green lush mountains. Nothing was familiar to me here. I am going to share more about Barb later.

My new home, church, and friends were a **part of God's plan** in healing my heart and much more!

36
CONVICTION

While teaching the youth of our church, these words hit me with deep conviction.

"The one who says he is in the Light and [yet] hates his brother [Christian,¹ born-again child of God his Father] is in darkness even until now. The one who loves and unselfishly seeks the best for his brother lives in the Light, and in him there is no occasion for stumbling or offense. But the one who hates (detests, despises) his brother [¹ in Christ] is in darkness and is walking (living) in the darkness and does not know where he is going because the darkness has blinded his eyes." (I John 2:9-11, Amplified Bible)

"Whoever says he is in the Light and hates his brother [in my case, my Mom] is in darkness even until now." It slammed me hard. I hated my mom because she was mentally ill. I am 580 miles away from her and still feel the effects of her illness.

According to these verses, was I walking in darkness? Was I blind? Did I not know where I was going? I didn't feel love for my mom, so was I a phony Christian? How could I be a youth leader? How could I even call myself a Christian? If I had believed in physically scourging myself, I would have put 30 lashes across my back. I cried out, *"Oh God, how can you use me? I have hatred in my heart! Please forgive me, God. Lord Jesus, heal me, I don't want to be in the darkness and not know where I am going. I want to love as you love, unconditionally."*

I called my dad to tell him Ken and I would be coming up to Washington State, and we would stay with him during our visit. "Mom might be coming home while you are here," Dad told me. I hung up the phone. In my mind I shouted, *I can't do this! I can't stay at my parents' house if Mom is home from the hospital!* Being released did not mean Mom was emotionally well. Panic shot through me like a bolt of electricity, as painful memories flooded in and started to wreak havoc with my emotions. When Mom was sick, I always had to walk on eggshells, never knowing how she would react to me or anyone else. I decided to call my dad back and tell him we wouldn't be staying at his place. *Surely Dad will understand,* I thought.

"Elaine, with My help you can do this. I will be with you; you are not alone," I heard God say to me.

"God, I don't trust You! I don't! I want to, but this is hard, God. It's so hard. I can't do this. Help me, I want to be healed!"

After I was done praying, I thought maybe I needed to call my pastor to tell him the truth about the hatred that was in me. It will be up to him if I am worthy to be a youth leader. I needed to get this out of me. I was so tired of living a lie. I didn't love God as I am to love.

I called the pastor and asked him to come over because I had a confession to make. I told Ken that the pastor was coming and that I wanted him to be present with me when the pastor arrived. "Why?" he asked.

"I will tell you when he gets here," I said, "I just want you to sit and listen." I needed my husband and my pastor to know about the real me!

I was ashamed of the hatred that I had kept hidden for so many years. I could not contain the truth of it any longer, even if the hatred didn't leave me.

The pastor arrived and sat in a chair opposite of Ken and myself. He knew a little about my mom's mental illness. "We are going to Washington soon and staying at my parents' house, and I don't think I can do it!" I blurted out.

"Why not?" he asked.

"I hate my mother," I spewed. "My heart is wicked! I am being eaten up on the inside by hatred. I won't blame you if you don't want me working with the youth anymore." With tears of anguish, the words poured out from me. The pastor and Ken sat there speechless. "Say something, I just poured out my guts!"

The pastor calmly leaned forward, his elbows on his knees and his hands under his chin. His eyes were gentle and in a soft voice, he asked me, "Elaine, do you really hate your mother?"

I looked at him, and in that moment, something profound took place in my heart. Truth stirred deep within me. "No," I said almost in a whisper, "but I hurt so badly! I love my mom, but it hurts." In the twinkling of an eye, God delivered me from the bondage of hatred, and I was free! God's indescribable peace came over me in that instant, and this was the beginning of my healing. A huge weight was lifted off and it was as though I could have floated off the couch. I sobbed tears of relief. For many years, I had been deceived into thinking the pain of having a mentally ill mother was the same as hatred.

Later, the pastor told me he really had no idea what to say to me in that moment of confession. I told him that God did, and God knew exactly what I needed to hear.

I sought the LORD, and He answered me, and delivered me from all my fears. (Psalm 34:4, English Standard Version)

Elaine Oostra

37
FACING MY FEARS

Ken and I drove to Washington State and made plans to stop at the hospital before we arrived at Dad's house. I no longer hated my mom, but I still feared going back into the hospital to see her. My heart became more anxious as we drew near.

These times were extremely difficult mentally, physically, and emotionally for us as a family. I would ask Dad how Mom was doing and all he could say was, "Mom is fine. I have it under control."

My dad started being more open with me about his struggles in dealing with a wife and son with mental illness. On one occasion, I was sitting in the car with Dad after visiting with Mom. He shared with me how hurtful it was when she threw her wedding ring at him and demanded a divorce. Dad knew she was not in her right mind, but this did not ease his pain. He felt rejected by the woman he loved.

Ken and I arrived at the hospital. We sat in the car, with dread. I was reluctant to go in. "We need to go in, but don't leave me," I said to Ken, "I can't do this without you." I took a deep breath to calm my pounding heart. *What will she be like?*

"God, please help me!" I prayed silently. We stepped out of the elevator onto the second floor into a small, colorless area with locked double doors and a phone on the wall. "I think we need to use this to get in," I said to Ken. "Hello? I am Elaine and I am here to see Joanne."

The nurse on the other end of the line replied, "I am sorry, visiting hours are not for another 30 minutes."

As I hung up the phone I wanted to scream, "Just let me in!" I had been emotionally prepared and now I have to do this again?

"Let's go and get some coffee," Ken said.

My internal anxiety would not let me sit. "I am going to walk around," I said to Ken.

Finally, the 30 minutes were over. I breathed deeply, trying to calm myself. I picked up the phone and identified myself, once again. The locked doors opened. We were immediately greeted by three nurses and handed clipboards asking for our personal information. Looking past the nurses and down the long hallway, I saw a small, white-haired, old woman. I handed my unfinished form to Ken and said, "Finish this for me, please."

"Mom? Mom?" Quickly I walked towards this woman. She looked at me. "Mom!" I began to cry uncontrollably. I grabbed her and pulled her to me. "Mom! Mom! Mom!" She looked up at me with no emotion, hands remaining at her side as if I should be the one committed. I didn't care. I had never been able to hug Mom when she was ill. Her mental illness had repulsed me but no longer. I felt true, unconditional love for her! Being in the mental hospital, a place I once hated, brought about an even deeper healing.

"Mom, show me your room." I took her hand and held it. I was giddy! Mom showed me the plastic, stained glass she had painted for each of her great-grandchildren. "Oh Mom, this is so sweet, thank you!"

"Here is a picture I colored," Mom said.

"Can I have it, Mom?" I asked. In her early 70's, Mom was

coloring from a child's book.

It was so sad to me, this place and why Mom was there, yet I knew it was best. My heart was overwhelmed sitting next to Mom on her bed. She had no clue of how God had healed me, let alone my struggles with her illness.

My Mom came home later that week. I looked in my parents' room to say good night on her first night home. I stood there, smiling. Dad was lying next to Mom with his arms wrapped around her, smiling from ear to ear. "Oh, how cute you two are!" I said. "Dad, don't you just love having Mom home?"

My dad hugged my unresponsive Mom even more and said, "Yep!"

"Well, I am going to leave you two lovebirds alone," I said to my parents. I went over to them and gave them a hug and a kiss good night. I was grinning like my dad, marveling in the grace of God over my life and the huge change in me.

A few years later, we were visiting Mom again in a different hospital. This place was more pleasant than the other hospitals. The staff was very caring. The room was more welcoming and with color on the walls, unlike the stark whiteness of previous facilities.

My younger brother and I were sitting next to Mom on the couch with our arms around her. She kept turning around looking out the window. It was dark outside.

"I need to go, he is following me," Mom said.

"Who is following you, Mom?" my brother and I both asked her.

"He is out there watching me," she said.

"Mom, no one is outside," I replied. We tried to assure her but to no avail.

"I have to go," she told us.

"Go where, Mom?"

"I can't tell you," Mom said. This conversation went on for a little while.

"Mom, where do you need to go?" I asked.

After much prompting and reassuring her she said, "I need to go to the river. I have to get rid of the snakes in my stomach. It's the only way to get rid of them."

My heart broke for her. I had never felt this sadness for her before. Instead, I had been focused on my own hurt.

I got up and went over to the nurses' station. "My mom wants to go to the river to get rid of the snakes, and this means Mom wants to go drown herself," I explained. We had gone through this many times before when we lived next to the river. The police would be called to hunt for Mom when she would wander off. I believe God's hand was on my mom's life to stop her from self-destructing during this awful time of illness. The nurse thanked me and then put a reclining chair in front of the nurses' station for Mom to sleep in so they could keep an eye on her.

"God, I don't understand all that Mom goes through with this illness, and why she has experienced all of this torment." It is a helpless feeling watching someone with mental illness fight unseen demons.

On our way back to Idaho, we stopped in to see Mom. I told Ken I wanted to go in by myself and say goodbye. I had some unfinished business to do. Mom was in bed, so I sat on her bed. She was doing much better. Taking my mom's hand, I said, "Mom, I need to tell you something and ask you something. I have been a horrible daughter to you. Could you forgive me?"

She looked at me, puzzled, "You have not been a horrible daughter. Why would you think that?"

"Mom, I have not been a good daughter. I know my heart." She reassured me again that she never thought I was a bad daughter. I was trying to hold back tears. What I saw was that my mom loved me and she didn't see the ugliness of my heart. She just loved me. It's the unconditional love of a parent. I was so glad that I, too, can love my mom back unconditionally. God did all this. He changed my heart, in His time and in His way.

I have been praying for many years for Mom to be free from mental and emotional illness. Mom is now in her 80's. The last few years have been very good, with only a few minor setbacks due to medications. I love my mom with all my heart. It's hard to leave her and Dad in my visits to Washington. I cry each time I leave. This is so opposite of how I used to feel. I know my time with them is short. I am so thankful for the relationship I have with my mom now. It's like God is restoring the years the locusts have eaten. I know He is!

Elaine Oostra

38
LIFE IN IDAHO

Being married to Kenny has lead me into a lot of new adventures. Most I would have never done or even thought of doing. When you are married to a farmer, you are definitely a 'help mate' whether you want to be or not.

Here I was in Idaho, in the dry desert. I saw so many allegories with irrigating and my growing faith. Being a Northwestern Washington girl, where the water comes from the sky, this irrigating thing was new to me. I learned fast that the only way to get our crop to grow was to water it. The water came from a reservoir, down the canals, though our main water line, then into our irrigation pipes and wheel lines, and finally onto the field through the sprinklers. Each of these sections have a valve to turn on or off for the water. Each needs to work properly to water the ground.

To me, God is like the reservoir. If we don't hook up to Him, we won't grow spiritually and learn to trust Him with every area of our lives. We need to turn the valves on in different areas for the water to flow, just as we do in our lives for spiritual growth. We will have issues if even the smallest valve malfunctions. God doesn't force us to change every area of our lives the minute we are saved any more than we dump the whole water reservoir on our fields. He takes it a section at a time and shows us broken valves. Water from a reservoir, through many processes, ends up coming out of a tiny sprinkler hole. This is how gentle God is with us in where we need to get rid of sin. There are no shortcuts in this process.

I had no clue how to milk a cow when we first had our dairy, even though I grew up on a farm. And I definitely had no clue how to irrigate. Yet, this had become my new job. I could write a separate book on my experiences on how NOT to farm. I had made every mistake there was to make, mainly because I did not enjoy milking or irrigating. However, if I had to pick, I would rather irrigate.

The years of working on our dairy taught me how to work hard. I am thankful for that. I also learned from my past struggles not to give up.

Here before me was a new challenge: how to hook up irrigation pipes and move wheel lines. My first time out in the fields that we rented, I must confess, I cried. I could not believe all the pipes that needed to be moved. I complained a lot. Again, this was not my plan for my life, but what made me think the world revolved around 'my plan'? You would think by this time I would know it's God that has a plan for my life. I did get into the routine of irrigating about five hay fields. It took me most of the day.

I want to tell you a funny story when I took a shortcut while irrigating. Well, it wasn't funny at the time. It reminds me of the mess I would make trying to fix things myself because I thought God was working too slowly.

One Sunday after church, I had to go out to a 100-acre field that we rented. It had about seven irrigating wheel lines I had to move. I really wanted to try hard and not get my hair wet. There was something at church later in the evening and I didn't want to have to do my hair over. Ken and I both went out to the field with his big, gray, diesel truck.

My job would be to hook the long, big hose back up to the wheel line, clamp the valve cap on the next rise, and turn the valve to release the seal cap inside of the riser. This allows the water to flow. The main water line is underground with the risers sticking out of the ground. The water pressure is like turning on a fire hydrant if the valve is wide open. Sound easy?

Nothing ever goes smoothly when you are in a hurry. It took me a long time of irrigating to understand this. Some of the valves in this field were buggers and made it hard to shut the water off. Since I was in a hurry, I parked Ken's truck in front of the next valve and hose that I had to move. I had the windows open in the truck as it was a hot day.

I turned the valve to shut off the water and could tell right away the seal inside was not where it was supposed to be, making it impossible to shut the water off. Shoot! This meant we had to shut down the main pump on the hill that feeds the main line. From afar, Ken saw I was having issues. With hand motions that I don't always understand from afar, he pointed to the hill where the main pump was. OK, common sense told me I had better wait for Ken. I knew it would take time to turn off the whole system and more time to start it all up again in order for the water to refill the main line.

I stood there looking at the valve. *I can do this.* I thought to myself with my still perfect, Sunday hair. *If I take the clamp off fast and screw the seal back in fast, we won't have to shut off everything.* Yet, my brain was screaming, "Wait for your husband!" Common sense did not win this argument inside of my brain. The illogical woman in me won.

I bent over above the valve, released the clamp, and WHAMP! The metal valve flew past my head, just missing me by maybe a fourth of an inch! Ken told me later, this could have killed me. A great force of water hit me in my face, and all I can think is, *MY HAIR!* I stood up in the middle of a waterfall pounding down around me. Have you ever stood in front of a fire hydrant going full board? Well, that is what it was like, except point the hydrant toward the sky.

I swam my way out. I was running out of breath. *The pickup!* I thought, as panic set it. I couldn't see because of all the falling water. I felt my way; I knew I had parked really close. Then I remembered, I had left the windows open! I found the truck door handle and pulled the door open. My plan was to start the truck as fast as I could and move it so that Ken wouldn't know I had parked that close. Yes, he had warned me about parking close to the valves. It really was a comical sight as I opened up the truck door and another river of water came pouring out. I made my way upstream into the truck and got it started with water still gushing in. I was attempting to take breaths of air. I moved it as fast as I could. I finally breathed.

I stopped the truck and got out to assess the damage I had made. Well, so much for Ken not noticing; a geyser of water shot into the air 100 feet. Water was still flowing from the open truck door and I was standing there, drenched, water dripping from my once perfect, Sunday hair, now pasted to my head. I looked out to the field. Ken was running toward me with his arms shaking in the air, meaning, "WHY?" I understood that look! Oh, boy, I had some explaining to do. Ken and I can laugh about this today.

My impatient behavior would not wait for my husband, who knew how to correctly handle the broken valve, which made it take longer to get the job done. I missed the church activity. We had to drive home in a very wet truck and oh, yes, my hair was ruined.

Sometimes I wish God would work faster in my life, but I have learned when I try to do things my way, I always make a bigger mess.

39
HAPPY 50TH SURPRISE!

God had torn down a lot of bricks since I was 28 from the wall that I built. Yet there were more bricks to go. God had healed the relationship with my mom; my marriage was next. This is a hard chapter for me to write, honestly. I want to respect my husband. I also am letting you know what a slow learner I am.

I know God has a sense of humor. He put man and woman together and said, "Get along!" Yet, He created male and female so differently. Then He said, "Woman, respect that man. Man, love that woman." This paraphrase is found in Ephesians chapter five. Read it for yourself. It's true!

God already knew wives would struggle to respect their husbands. He knew husbands would have a hard time loving their wives. Men tend to turn to their work, sports, and hobbies, then without a clue, neglect their wives. Women struggle respecting their husbands when they see that "the prince on the white horse" that courted them now has tons of flaws and it's her job, she feels, to point them out. Husbands forget God made them to be the spiritual leaders of the home and women forget they were created to come alongside their men, not to usurp them and lord over them. This is in I Timothy chapter two. God said all this, not me!

I was married to a man, who thought, talked, and walked like a no-nonsense type of man. There also was a downside to this macho man. My man did not want to read or study anything, especially on how to better your marriage. He loved me and that was good enough.

Romance is a word that is very foreign to my type of man. A gift will be something you need, like a new shovel for the barn. OK, I will give him credit. As many years went on, Ken gave me more personal gifts. Was it maybe something I said?

I will be honest, I was not content with my type of man. He resisted me anytime I tried to tell him where I felt he needed to change. Imagine that.

I became very discontent and found myself building a wall to isolate myself from him. I don't even know if he noticed. As long as I was there and food was on the table, he was content.

Divorce was not an option for me, because I saw the love my dad had for my mom in spite of all the hardships he went through with her. Yet, why did I think treating my husband coldly was OK? It was like God hit me over the head with a two by four. I was convicted. I saw the enemy's plot toward my marriage. I saw the lies the enemy was trying to get me to believe. I cried out to God, repented, and asked Him to change me. **Psalm 51:12** became my prayer, **"Restore unto me the joy of Your salvation And sustain me with a willing spirit." (New American Standard Bible)**

Meanwhile, unbeknownst to me, my husband was planning a party for my 50th birthday. He also was planning another big event.

I was working in the backyard when I looked up and saw my dearest friend from Washington walking toward me! "What are you doing here? How?" I excitedly asked her.

"Your husband invited me to spend your birthday with you!" she told me.

"This is amazing!" I said. I couldn't believe he had done this.

A couple of days later my mom, dad, and one of my daughters with my granddaughter showed up from Washington!

"Let's have a girl's day for your birthday, Mom," my daughter said.

"I would like us girls to go to the gift shop for a latte and then go shopping," I suggested.

I fell perfectly into Ken's plot. He knew me!

I walked into the gift shop and the owner, my friend, had all these tables set up with tons of food arranged very nicely. Some of my friends were there. "Wow, are you having a party or something?" I asked her.

Then I heard it. "SURPRISE!" Some of Ken's sisters, his parents, and my other granddaughter came in! My niece, my sister, and brother arrived. They were all from Washington. I couldn't believe my husband had done this!

I was so pleased when I found out everyone was going to church on Sunday with us before they left to go back to Washington. At our church, when you have a birthday or anniversary, you go up front and the pastor prays over you. Our anniversary was just a few days away. I whispered to Ken, "Will you go up front with me for prayer?"

"Oh, I suppose so," he said roughly.

I was thrilled! He had never done this before, and had made it clear in the past he never would stand up in front of people.

We told the new pastor this was our 33rd wedding anniversary. After the prayer, I walked down the aisle toward my seat when, from the corner of my eye, I noticed Ken had put on a suit coat. I thought, *In the heat of June?* The pastor then asked me where I was going. "Um, to my seat?"

"You need to come up front," he said to me. I stood there clueless. *Why does Ken have a flower on his lapel?* "Elaine, come up," the pastor said again. "Weeks ago, Ken asked me if I would officiate in renewing their vows," the pastor told the congregation and me. "He told me you did not get married in the church, so he wants to do this right."

"He did?" I asked the pastor, then quickly grabbed my husband around the neck, hugging him. Tears filled my eyes. "You did this for me, for us? You planned ALL this?" My unromantic husband had done this! There was even a bride's bouquet of roses for me to hold!

Many of the people in the pews, now standing, were crying and clapping. They knew my man! They knew he is a man's man and not a romantic. Some people told me later that if so and so would have done this, it would have been no big deal, predictable even. Some of the guys who were like Ken, said, "Thanks Ken, for showing us up. How are we supposed to top that?"

The day before, my daughters had tricked me into buying a new outfit just for this occasion. They really wanted me to have a white top. Now I knew why!

As we were getting ready to say our vows, my dad pops up from his pew, "I never got to walk her down a church aisle!" The pastor told my dad to come up and get his daughter and walk her down. My dad did, smiling proudly all the way.

Never in a million years did I ever see my husband doing this, ever! I saw that day, for the first time, the love Ken had for me. I was the one who resisted it.

He still is his gruff self, and I am still me. I am learning to love him unconditionally as he is me. Isn't this the love God wants us to learn? And what a perfect way to teach us, through marriage. Like I said, I think God has a sense of humor.

We still have our struggles. We still argue. We call it communicating. We get it out and then we are fine.

Things that used to seem so big to me in our marriage and make me upset now seem so piddly. It's part of growing old together.

I am so thankful our kids have their parents together. Till death do us part is the promise we made and we are sticking to it!

Again, I want to make a tribute to my parents and their marriage and to my dad's faithfulness to my mom. He meant what he said, "In sickness and in health, till death do us part." I saw their love for each other, imperfect as it was and full of many trials and tribulations. *"Thank you, God for the example you set before Ken and me of what unconditional love looks like. I pray we are this to our kids and grandkids, imperfect as Ken and I are. But we serve a perfect God!"*

"Therefore, my beloved, be steadfast, immovable, always abounding in the work of the Lord, knowing that your toil is not in vain in the Lord." (I Corinthians 15:58 NASB)

Elaine Oostra

40
MY TRIBUTE TO MY FRIEND, BARB

One day, I was getting my hair foiled. Yep, that's tin foil all over my head that somehow holds the color product. What I won't go through to cover those gray hairs I am not ready to show to the world yet. Vain, I know.

In walked a young man I had in youth group several years before. I don't know about you, but I really don't like others, especially males, seeing me sitting in that chair looking like someone from outer space. I was held captive by my own hair with no way to escape! He sat down, not understanding how awkward this was for me. Finally, I told him I didn't like him seeing me like this. He replied back that it didn't matter to him. *Ok*, I thought, *get over yourself.*

As we started to chat, I saw and heard how much he needed to talk about issues in his life. He trusted the hairdresser and me with his heart. At one point, I even told him to tell me to be quiet if I was saying too much. He said, "No, I want to hear what you have to say." He was hurting.

I still can't believe that I was sitting in that chair looking like an antenna had blown up on my head, ministering to this young man. My poor hairdresser had to keep grabbing my head as I wanted eye contact with him. She warned me it would be my fault if the color and cut were uneven.

The next morning, I was thanking my Father in Heaven for bringing me to this little town that I had never heard of. I thought of the opportunity God had given to me while getting my hair cut. Also earlier in the day, I had led a Bible study with young moms and another study with teens. My thoughts immediately went to an amazing woman God placed in my life and all I had learned from her.

As I told you, I moved to Parma grudgingly. I had prayed for God to bring friends into my life. I struggled in making new friends and hated to leave a dear friend who knew me well. I was leaving my security of everything and everyone I knew.

Sitting behind Barb the first Sunday we showed up at the new church, I knew I wanted to get to know that woman! She turned around with her face lit up and radiating Christ and grabbed my hand to welcome me. God definitely had a plan. How do I put on paper the last 17 years of knowing this amazing woman and all I have learned from her?

Before I knew Barb, the thought of ministering to other people was scary to me. I would do it only in a safe environment, like church. When I hung out with Barb, I watched in amazement how she reached out to people anywhere. I saw her take strangers into her home. Through her, I met people I thought I would never associate with. I saw things in myself I didn't like. Barb cared about other people's lives and what got them into their particular situations. She listened! She loved unconditionally.

Without even knowing it, I was job shadowing her. God was teaching me and growing me. There is a verse about the older women teaching the younger women. I wanted God to use me as a woman to teach the younger. This became more and more the desire of my heart as I watched Barb. I would kid and tell others, "When I grow up I want to be like Barb." I knew there was only one Barb in this world, but I was finding myself doing some of the same things I admired so much in her. Oh, that I could be this example to other young women! Barb and I had our differences in some Biblical nonessentials, but in the essentials, we very much agreed. I have always felt such unconditional love from Barb. I had that for her as well.

She knew my struggles with my mom and was a big part in my healing process. I could tell Barb anything and she would not be shocked. My favorite thing she would say to me was "We need to pray about this," and we would. She was a huge encourager and has been with me step by step in the healing process of my past pain. I know that I am spiritually stronger than I was almost 17 years ago. God used her mightily in my life.

I have felt, in a sense, like a bird kicked out of the nest ready to fly on her own. I have felt this the last couple of years, knowing God would change our relationship by moving her away. A few months ago (July, 2015), she and her husband moved miles away to be with their grandkids, a dream come true for Barb.

Thank you, Barb, for the Jesus Christ I see in you! I still have so much to learn in ministering to others. I did learn I can minister even with an explosion of tin foil on my head! God knew when I moved 580 miles who I was going to meet. He knew what work He needed to do in me. He knew just the person He wanted to use in my life. Yes, there have been others too, but I know my life wouldn't be the same today without you in it. I love you Barb!

Dear Elaine,

I am so grateful for this tribute! Maybe you can read it at my memorial service! Lol! Life would have been so boring here in Parma these past many years without you to watch and encourage. I feel like you have had to go through all the trials while I sat on the sidelines and cheered you on, but I surely have watched you victoriously overcome! I think I have learned more from you, Sweetpea!!! But thanks anyway! I love you too, Elaine!

Barb

Elaine Oostra

41
CONCLUSION

On a recent trip to Washington, Ken and I went to the rest home to see his mom. Walking down the hallway, I looked at the names and pictures of people occupying the rooms. Next to Ken's mom's room were my old neighbors, Jerry and Sandra (not real names) who took care of me when my mom was sick. I entered their room hesitantly, "Are you Sandra?"

"Yes," she replied back.

"Do you know who I am?" I asked her as I bent down close to her. She looked at me with a puzzled look. I was not sure how her memory was. "I am Elaine, I was your neighbor, and you took care of me when I was a child." I said to her.

A look of recognition came into her eyes and a smile appeared on her face. "Yes, I remember you! It's been a long time." I sat on her bed. She was sitting in her chair. We chatted about the past. Forgotten were the hard times I had as a little girl away from home and staying with them. I looked into the eyes of this elderly woman; at 93, her mind was pretty good. I felt great respect for her.

"I remember one day when your dad dropped off your sister; she was a baby. He didn't ask, he just brought her over." Sandra told me.

"Was my mom sick? I wonder where the rest of us were," I asked.

"She must have been. Your dad had to work on the farm and he couldn't with a baby. So he just brought her over, knowing I would take her. When the corn was high, your mom would go down all the rows of corn and hide from your dad," Sandra said.

Jerry wheeled into the room with his wheelchair. His mind was not as good as Sandra's. I asked him if he remembered me. I tried, unsuccessfully, a few times to jolt his memory. Sandra and I were chatting when he looked at his wife and said, "She looks like Eileen." (I get called Eileen a lot).

I got up and grabbed his hands, "It's me Jerry, Elaine! You took care of me!"

He looked puzzled and again he looked at his wife of 73 years, "She sure looks like Eileen."

I put my hands on my face and again said, "It's me!" After doing this a few more times, I think he got it. Well, for a little while.

"We need to go home, I have to milk the cows," Jerry said.

Sandra gave him a look I remember as a child when she would be a little frustrated at Jerry for falling asleep at the table, praying. It made me smile knowing God purposely put Jerry and Sandra right next to my mother-in-law.

I love how God brings things full circle. Things that were hard in childhood were now healed. Still at times, God heals even more. I love this about God!

I still am amazed at the transformation God did in me because I kept crying out to Him. I will continue to do this in each trial I face. God is faithful! I know this now. I hope in reading my story, you are encouraged to put all your pain and hurt in His care one brick at a time, to put each day into His hands, and to put on humility and take off pride. Pride has to hide things in our past.

Humility frees us.

Just as when others write their life stories, the end of the book is really not the end. There is more to be said. Life goes on. My dad has dementia and is living in a health care center. I have to put in a code to his hall. It's like the roles between my parents have been reversed. My mom is living in a resident care home and at this time doing pretty well. The part of life where our parents age is another whole story. It's difficult.

Healing goes on until we are in heaven with our Savior. Life continues to have trials; the Bible says not to be surprised at them. God uses them to perfect us for that day that we will stand before Him, rejoicing and not be ashamed. Trials empty us of ourselves and fill us up with Christ's likeness. God is sovereign, always. Suffering always leads to freedom and adversity frees us from the bondage we live under. My life testifies of this. I am free! My chains are gone!

Elaine Oostra

42
SELF REFLECTIONS

There may still be a layer of bricks at my feet that needs to be torn away. Maybe it's just to remind me to remain humble and have empathy for others. Maybe it's so I will know God's grace is always sufficient for me. I know I no longer want to add more bricks and when one comes, usually in the form of pride, I cry out to God, *"Search my heart and see if there be any wicked way in me!"*

I am continually working on relationships, asking God to show me my part if something has gone askew. I can't change others, but I can change me.

In my story, I talked about having a bitterroot grow. I want to help you understand what a bitterroot looks like. In italics are personal questions you can ask yourself.

When I read Jim Wilson's book, *How to be Free from Bitterness,* some of these facts hit me hard. I came to recognize when I would allow this bitterroot to take hold of my life and allow it to grow. I was a child when I planted that bitter seed and determined that no one was going to hurt me anymore. The bitter seed came in the form of a wall of self-protection.

Do you know when the bitterroot started in you? What does yours look like? How has it disguised itself? You may not see it right away. Keep this question in the back of your mind as you continue to read.

I knew I could not change what I did not acknowledge. When I repented and confessed my bitterness as a sin against God, I experienced forgiveness and joy. Being free from bitterness for me took time. Old habits are hard to break, BUT they will be broken when you ask God to change your old way of thinking and don't give up.

I am going to share with you some Bible verses from the New International Version to understand bitterroots because I believe God and His Word are the only way to be cured of them.

I am going to define a Biblical bitterroot.
"See to it that no one falls short of the grace of God and that no bitter root grows up to cause trouble and defile many." (Hebrews 12:15, NIV)

Bitterness is a root. It is something you can't see because it's underground, but there is visible evidence of a root. We have seen the damage tree roots do to a sidewalk or to my sewer tile line in my back yard. I can't see those roots, but I know they have grown into my tile when the waste from my house backs up. This root sprung up and caused trouble and defiled my shower drain. When bitterness comes out of us, it defiles others.

Do you recognize people you lash out at or can't stand to be around?

How do I know if I have a bitterroot?
Bitterness remembers details; review, review, and review. You can't remember a single happy moment. You only see how right you are and how wrong everyone else is. It causes you to only see what the offender did, causing feelings of hatred, jealousy, resentment, and envy. Other people make you mad,

even though they don't have that power over you. It's your choice, yet you blame them.

Bitterness is what we feel when *others* sin against us. Bitterness is related to those who are close to us. Guilt is what we feel when *we* sin.

Do you remember every detail of how someone hurt you years ago? Do you remind them every chance you get?

Can others see my bitterroot?

Yes! It's seen in the eyes and in the lines of the face. You can see it in our mouths when we are smiling. You can hear it in the tone of a voice.

Do you find yourself glaring at those who hurt you? Do you put on a fake smile? Are you sarcastic or do you excuse what you said by saying, "I was only kidding"?

What does the Bible teach about the bitterroot?

"But if you harbor bitter envy and selfish ambition in your hearts, do not boast about it or deny the truth. Such "wisdom" does not come down from heaven but is earthly, unspiritual, and demonic. For where you have envy and selfish ambition, there you find disorder and every evil practice." (James 3:14, 16, NIV)

How does the Bible teach us to get rid of the bitterroot? What is God's solution for my bitterroot?

Dig it up! Get rid of it. This takes the grace of God. It takes knowing Jesus Christ to be able to do this. He is the source of grace.

"Get rid of all bitterness, rage and anger, brawling and slander, along with every form of malice. Be kind and compassionate to one another, forgiving each other, just as in Christ God forgave you. Follow God's example, therefore, as dearly loved children and walk in the way of love, just as Christ loved us and gave himself unto for us as a fragrant offering and sacrifice to God." (Ephesians 4:31 – 5:2, NIV)

What do I do with my bitterroot?

You can keep the bitterness in and make yourself sick or let it out and spread the sickness around. Neither way is God's way, but it's what people do.

Bitterness is my sin regardless of what I think caused it. It's what we do and what we are. What people do to us only spills out what is in us. If we are sweet, sweet water will spill out. If we are bitter, bitter water will spill out. We must get rid of it and not share it. We need to see it for what it is, evil. It's not gone by someone saying they are sorry. It doesn't disappear even if this person dies.

When we confess our sins and understand God's forgiveness for ourselves, we will be able to forgive others. We can only give out the grace to others that we have received from God.

When people ruffle your feathers, how do you react? What comes out: bitter or sweet?

How do I forgive others so I don't let this root grow?

"This is how my heavenly Father will treat each of you unless you forgive your brother or sister from your heart." (Matthew 18:35, NIV)

Do not take revenge, my dear friends, but leave room for God's wrath, for it is written: "It is mine to avenge; I will repay," says the Lord." (Romans 12:19, NIV)

Are you of the mindset that if you forgive the person, you are letting them off the hook for what they did? Do you trust God to repay?

How many times do I forgive?

"I tell you, not seven times, but seventy-seven times." (Matthew 18:22, NIV)

Jesus knows the other person has sinned against you, but if we are counting, then we are not forgiving.

When I was born again, God unconditionally forgave me. So I must unconditionally forgive.

"And forgive us our debts, as we have also forgiven our debtors." (Matthew 6:12, NIV)

"for if you forgive men when they sin against you, your heavenly Father will forgive you, BUT if you do not forgive other people of their sins, your Father will not forgive your sins." (Matthew 6:14, NIV)

People know when we really come to them with a forgiving heart when they have hurt you. It doesn't mean you will always win them over. We can only go to the person when there is forgiveness in our own hearts. **Forgiveness is not dependent on the other person's repentance.**

Do you only want to forgive so the other person will repent?

As a forgiven Christian, who has forgiveness from the heart, I need to be concerned about the person who did the sinning against me. I can't or won't be concerned about myself. Real forgiveness does not keep a record of wrongs. I can't have unforgiveness in my heart and still rejoice in the Lord.

Are you able yet to be concerned about the person who hurt you and why they did it and what is going on in their hearts?

One of my favorite verses in the bible is **Psalm 139:23-24 "Search me, O God, and know my heart; test me and know my anxious thoughts. See if there is any offensive way in me, and lead me in the way of everlasting." (NIV)**

When I start to feel anger or bitterness toward someone, I cry out this prayer. I know where bitterness leads and I don't want to go down that road again. If you read the verses above 23 and 24, you will see David was angry and hated his enemy. Somehow this brings me comfort, knowing David struggled like I do, and he knew to Whom he should turn.

The bitterroot takes offense.

Have you ever said, "I am not bitter, I just get easily hurt."

Did you know the symptoms of getting hurt easily are close to the symptoms of resentment? You get hurt and take offense, holding onto the offense until it rots. It's caused some to commit murder.

Do you recognize that this stops you from sincerely forgiving?

Again, a person can apologize to you until they are blue in the face, but it will NOT get rid of bitterness and an offense in the heart. The ONLY solution for those easily hurt, those who take up an offense, is to confess this before God because of what Jesus Christ did for us on the cross, dying for our sins and rising again.

Can you do this, or will pride keep your mind on the offender and not your own sin?

"Have this attitude in yourselves which was also in Christ Jesus who, although He existed in the form of God, did not regard equality with God a thing to be grasped, but emptied Himself, taking the form of a bondservant and being made in the likeness of men. Being found in appearance as a man, He humbles Himself by becoming obedient to the point of death, even death on a cross." (Philippians 2:5-8, New American Standard Bible)

We can't hold onto our identity and rights. We need to empty ourselves, be a servant, and be humble as Christ was.

Do you think about the lack of love in the other person and how he needs help, or are you thinking how the lack of love in the other person affects you? Read what I Corinthians 13 says about love.

Bitterness stops us from respecting those God calls us to respect.

When I was a youth leader, I had a teen boy in the group who came from a very rough background. I was teaching on the Ten Commandments and that week was "Honor your father and your mother." This teen angrily said to me, "I cannot and will not honor and respect my parents. They don't deserve it."

I knew his background. Did he have a right to say this? Yes. My challenge was to teach him to let go of that right.

I told him he needed to respect their position in his life as parents, meaning their title. I also told him to be careful with hate. You become what you hate.

If I don't care for the President of the United States because of his policies, I still need to respect his position as our president.

Have you found yourself holding back respect from those God called you to respect: a parent or a boss? A wife is called by God to respect her husband. As a wife, are you not respecting your husband because you feel he doesn't deserve it? (Love and Respect by John Eldridge is a great book)

How do I turn bitterness into love?
"But where sin increased, grace increased all the more." (Romans 5:20b, NIV)

"Be kind and compassionate to one another, forgiving each other, just as in Christ God forgave you." (Ephesian 4:32, NIV)

We need to, we must, surrender our bitterness to God and

allow God's grace to fill us. The Holy Spirit will do this in us. Cry out to Him! I have done this many times when I have struggled with bitterness. I confessed it out loud even. I cried out to God to help me to love and forgive. Sometimes I didn't even understand why I had bitterness. I did know, however, that I could tell God all about it and He would listen. He would change my heart. I couldn't do it.

I started to see the person or situation differently, I would see their pain and what caused them to treat others poorly. My eyes were off myself. I still live in the fleshly body and struggle with sin, but Jesus Christ has given me a way out of each temptation that I face. I can go to my Heavenly Father and sit before His throne. Repentance through Jesus has made this possible. As dirty as I see myself with my sin before me, my Heavenly Father sees me clean and pure, as white as snow!

This is how God wants me to see others: as He sees me, loved and forgiven. When I forgive others and love them, I pray it will lead them to Jesus Christ if they don't know Him.

Because God has forgiven me much, much is required of me to forgive others. If I don't forgive others, I will not be forgiven. This is a huge motivator to forgive!

My hope and my prayer is that through my story you will understand God's unlimited love for you. If you are a believer in Jesus Christ, I hope you see you are not the only one who has struggles with anger, bitterness and rage. God heals us of these things when we continue to cry out to Him until He changes us. Persevere! God will deliver you! Humble yourselves before Him and walk in obedience to Him.

If you are not a believer in the saving grace of Jesus Christ, no matter how hard you try, the human nature is prone to sin. You can't get rid of it. It can only be done by God. We are all born with a sin nature. We see it in babies on up. We demand our way. We cry when we don't get our way. We are selfish and self-centered. This is what sin is. We put ourselves first and on the throne of our lives. Like one of my daughters would say when she was two years old, " I do myself!" Let me share some main points with you if you want or need to be set free from guilt, bitterness, fits of rage, or other things in your life.

1. You need to know you are helpless to change this in yourself.

2. Being 'good' does not set you free. The Bible tells us that none of us are good! Our thought life alone would condemn us!

3. You need to know and believe that God already accomplished the work to set you free through Jesus's death on the cross.

"You see, at just the right time, when we were still powerless, Christ died for the ungodly." (Romans 5:6, NIV)

"But God demonstrated his own love for us in this: While we were still sinners, Christ died for us." (Romans 5:8, NIV)

"He was delivered over to death for our sins and was raised to life for our justification." (Romans 4:25, NIV)

God doesn't ask you to change first. He takes you as you are! He took me.

4. God, through the Holy Spirit, will draw you to Himself. He will give you the desire to call on the name of Jesus, and trust Him.

5. **"If you declare with your mouth, 'Jesus is Lord,' and believe in your heart that God raised Him from the dead, you will be saved. (11)Anyone who believes in him will never be put to shame." (Romans 10:9,11, NIV)** What a wonderful promise!

6. Thank God for forgiving you and giving you Eternal Life.
If you have given your life over to Jesus Christ, to have him reign over your life, please tell someone. You can email me at fieldofviewpress@gmail.com . Find a Bible-believing church.

There are many churches that don't believe what the Word of God says. Ask God to lead you to the right place and people. Start reading the Bible and possibly attend a Bible study. If you now have a new life in Christ, I would love to hear about it!

43
Dad

As I am finishing up the editing part of this book, my precious dad went to be with Jesus. I never got the chance to tell him about this book. I know he would have been proud of me. He left his health care residence and entered into his final residence, his heavenly mansion on March 28, 2016.

This is the Psalm his children chose for his service.

1 "I lift up my eyes to the hills. From where does my help come?

2 My help comes from the Lord, who made heaven and earth.

3 He will not let your foot be moved; he who keeps you will not slumber.

4 Behold, he who keeps Israel will neither slumber nor sleep.

5 The Lord is your keeper; the Lord is your shade on your right hand.

6 The sun shall not strike you by day, nor the moon by night.

7 The Lord will keep you from all evil; he will keep your life.

8 The Lord will keep your going out and your coming in from this time forth and forevermore." (Psalm 121:1-8 English Standard Version)

My dad loved the hills, he loved the mountains, he loved hiking. It was a refreshing relief from the trials of life. My dad served the Creator, not creation.

These were the words we came up with to describe our dad: honest, servant, faithful, diligent, integrity, a man of character, loving, funny, jokester, hardworking, doer of faith, awesome picture of unconditional love, and many more words.

"Blessed is the man who remains steadfast under trial, for when he has stood the test he will receive the crown of life, which God has promised to those who love him." (James 1:12, ESV)

"You see that faith was active along with his works, and faith was completed by his works." (James 2:22, ESV)

"Not only that, but we rejoice in our sufferings, knowing that suffering produces endurance, [4] and endurance produces character, and character produces hope, [5] and hope does not put us to shame, because God's love has been poured into our hearts through the Holy Spirit who has been given to us." (Romans 5:3-5, ESV)

Just a month before dad passing, I was in Washington. It was the last time I saw my dad alive. The night before Ken and I headed back to Idaho, we stopped at the health care center to say goodbye. Ken went to his mom's room and I went to my dad's. My dad had dementia; he still knew who we were and where he was. Yet, he had times of confusion and agitation. This was hard for him and hard for his family.

I tucked my dad into his bed, telling him I was leaving for Idaho and not sure when I was coming back, but would try to make it back soon. We hugged and kissed.

My dad was really awkward at I love you's, but I have never doubted his love for me! I headed down the hallway, almost reaching the doors to leave, when I heard, "Elaine ! Elaine!" I turned around and my dad was walking quickly down the hall toward me, arms waving in the air. "Elaine, I need to say goodbye before you go!" my dad excitedly said. I smiled. When he reached me, he put his arms around me, and I put mine around him. I gave him one more kiss and he returned one to me. The cleaning lady was standing near us when my dad told her, "This is my daughter!"

I know I am loved, I know he is proud of me. "Dad, I love you!" I told him. I waved at my dad as he walked back to his room. Tears came to my eyes and I wondered if it would be the last time I would see him. It was. *Thank you, Heavenly Father for this last wonderful memory with my dad! I know he is in heaven and I will see him again! Yet, my heart mourns the loss on this earth of holding him one more time. Yet! My heart rejoices because he is free!*

I said it before, but it is worth repeating and fits even more with the passing of my dad. Healing goes on till we are in heaven with our Savior. Life continues to have trials; the Bible says not to be surprised at them. God uses them to perfect us for that day that we will stand before Him, rejoicing and not be ashamed. Trials empty us of ourselves and fill us up with Christ's likeness. God is sovereign, always. Suffering always leads to freedom and adversity frees us from the bondage we live under. My life testifies of this. I am free! My chains are gone!

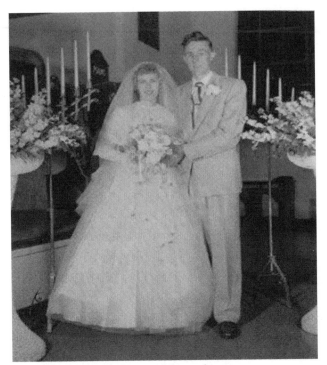

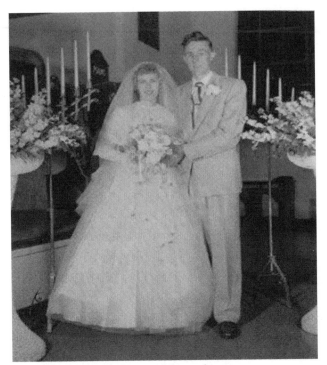

My mom and dad's wedding day.

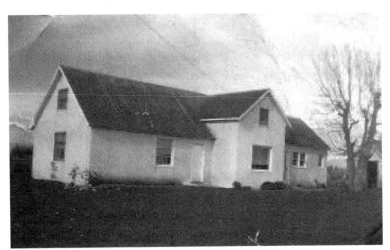

The old farmhouse.

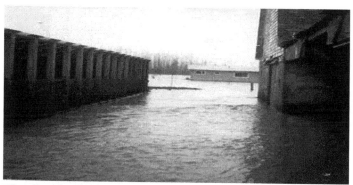

The floods cleaning out the barn.

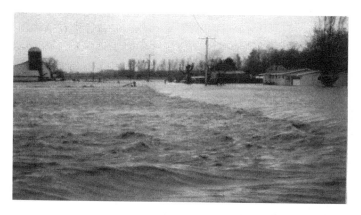

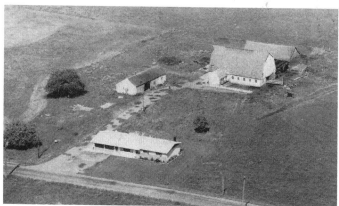

The farm where I grew up. The old farmhouse was between the trees.

Elaine Oostra

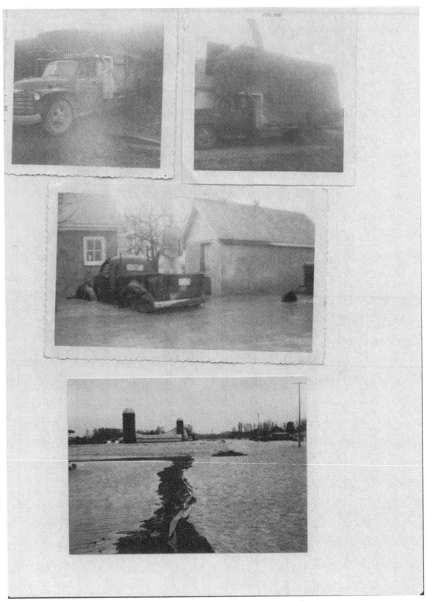

Silage truck and flooding by our house.

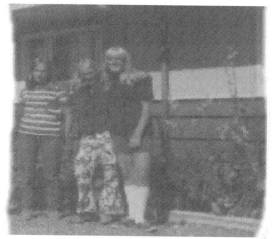

Childhood friends.

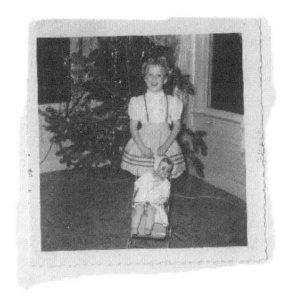

Me standing by my grandma's Christmas tree.

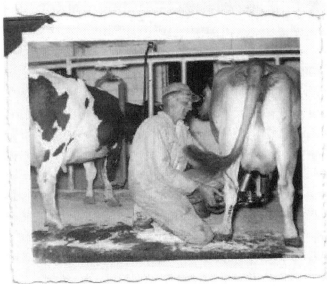

My dad milking in the stanchion barn.

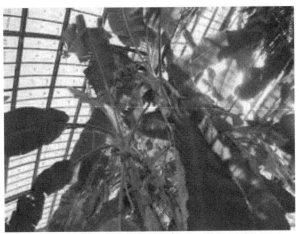

What the skylight looked like with the banana tree.

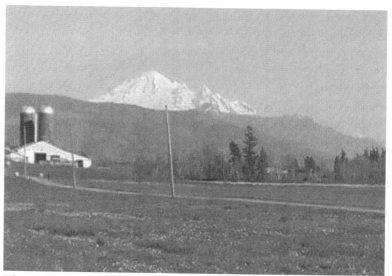

The mountains near where I grew up.

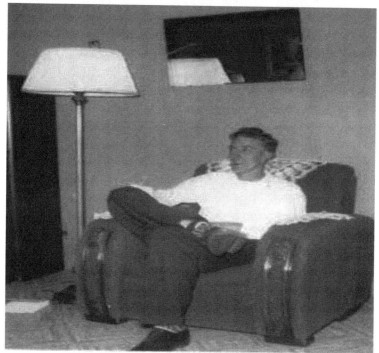

My dad in the chair from my first memory.

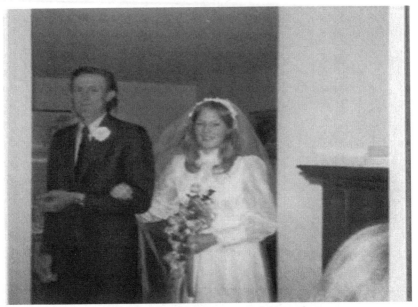

My dad and I on my wedding day.

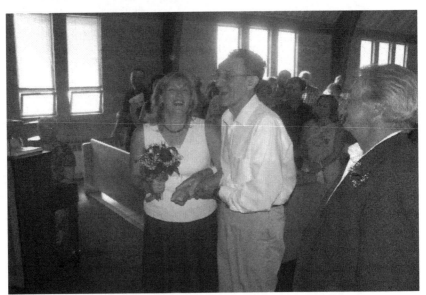

My dad telling the pastor he never got to walk me down a church aisle.

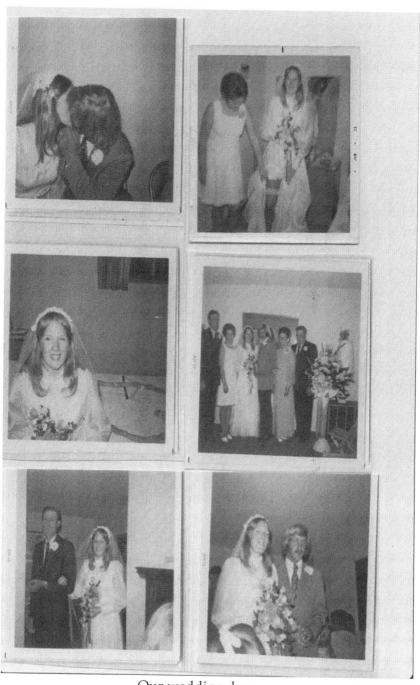

Our wedding day.

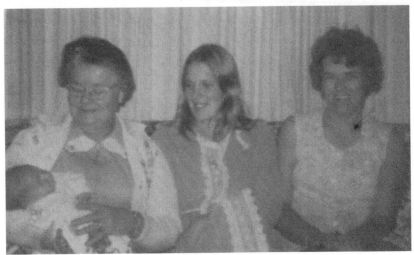

My grandmother, my first baby, myself and my mom.

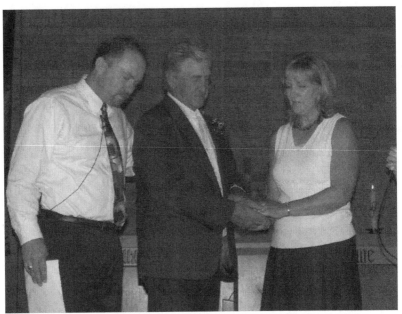

Ken surprised me with renewing our vows in church.

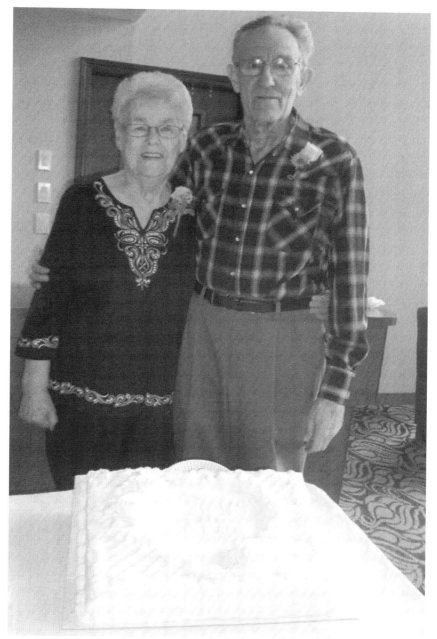

Celebrating 60 years of faithfulness to each other!

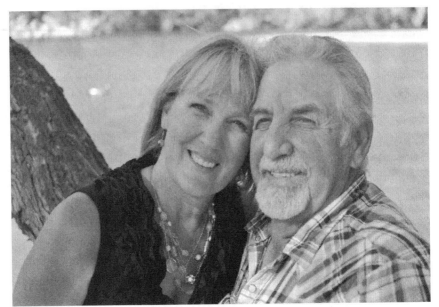

40 years together!

BIBLIOGRAPHY

Wilson, J., How To Be Free From Bitterness by Jim Wilson Community Christian Ministries http://www.ccmbooks.org

Bourasaw, N., 2003, History of Northern State Hospital of Sedro-Woolley, Washington, http://www.skagitriverjournal.com/NearbyS-W/NSH/NSH1-Intro.html

Deinstitutionalization: A Psychiatric Titanic, Frontline. Article from the Appendix of: out of the Shadows: Confronting America's Mental Illness Crisis. Torrey, E. Fuller M.D., New York, John Wiley & Sons, 1997 http://www.pbs.org/wgbh/pages/frontline/shows/asylums/special/excerpt.html

Diagnostic criteria for Schizophrenia; Schizophrenia.com http://schizophrenia.com/ami/diagnosis/mrBIPOL.html#common

Kruckenberg, S. (September 5, 2012) LPS Act - California Hospital Association,Lanterman-Petris-Short Act - Involuntary Commitment Act of 1967 http://www.bing.com/search?q=Lanterman+Petris+Short+LPS+Act&FORM=QSRE1

Crabb, L , Inside Out, Colorado Springs, CO, Navpress Publishing Group, 1998 Print

Dr Emerson Eggerichs, Love and Respect, Integrity Publishers, 2004, Print

Swindoll, Charles R., Strike the Original Match, Multnomah, 1980, First published: November 1981 Print

Beattie, Melody, Codependent No More, Hazelden Publishing, Center City, MN 1986 (first edition)

ABOUT THE AUTHOR

Elaine Oostra is the author of One Brick at a Time: Breaking Down the Wall of Bitterness and Learning to Trust God. She has studied the Bible for 20 years through Precept Ministries, an in-depth Bible class. It prepared her for what God had in store for her. Elaine serves in different youth ministries, including Launch Pad Ministries, a Christian release time class for middle and high school students. She has also served as a youth leader for nine years in her church. For the past 13 years, she has had and continues to have Bible studies in her home for high school girls. God has given her a passion and gift for teaching the youth.

Elaine and her husband have been married for 43 years (2016) and are self-employed farmers. They have four children, and four in-law(love) children, 15 grandchildren and 5 step grandchildren that are the delights of their hearts!

The joy of her heart is to see ALL come to a saving knowledge of Jesus Christ.

One Brick at a Time

Made in the USA
Charleston, SC
22 May 2016